AF348829

Cancer Treatment and Research

Volume 155

Series Editor
Steven T. Rosen

For further volumes:
http://www.springer.com/series/5808

Boris Pasche
Editor

Cancer Genetics

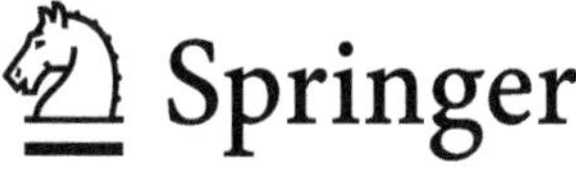 Springer

Editor
Boris Pasche, MD, PhD, FACP
The UAB Comprehensive Cancer Center
Division of Hematology/Oncology
The University of Alabama at Birmingham
Birmingham, AL, USA
boris.pasche@ccc.uab.edu

ISSN 0927-3042
ISBN 978-1-4419-6032-0   e-ISBN 978-1-4419-6033-7
DOI 10.1007/978-1-4419-6033-7
Springer New York Dordrecht Heidelberg London

Library of Congress Control Number: 2010927443

Printed on acid-free paper

Springer is part of Springer Science+Business Media (www.springer.com)

Contents

Contributors

Naresh Bellam Division of Hematology/Oncology, Department of Medicine, UAB Comprehensive Cancer Center, The University of Alabama, Birmingham, AL 35294-3300, USA

Mario Capasso CEINGE Advanced Biotechnologies, University of Naples "Federico II", Naples, Italy

Sharon J. Diskin Oncology Division, Center for Childhood Cancer Research, The Children's Hospital of Philadelphia, Philadelphia, PA 19104, USA

Diana Eccles Human Genetics and Cancer Sciences Divisions, School of Medicine, University of Southampton, Southampton University Hospitals NHS Trust, SO16 6YD, UK

David Huntsman Department of Pathology and Laboratory Medicine, Vancouver General Hospital, University of British Columbia, British Columbia Cancer Agency, Vancouver, BC, Canada V5Z 4E6

Kenneth Offit Clinical Genetics Service, Memorial Sloan-Kettering Cancer Center, New York, NY 10021, USA

Boris Pasche Division of Hematology/Oncology, Department of Medicine, UAB Comprehensive Cancer Center, The University of Alabama, Birmingham, AL 35294-3300, USA

Kasmintan Schrader Department of Pathology and Laboratory Medicine and Department of Medical Genetics, University of British Columbia, British Columbia Cancer Agency, Vancouver, BC, Canada V5Z 4E6

William Tapper Human Genetics and Cancer Sciences Divisions, School of Medicine, University of Southampton, Southampton University Hospitals NHS Trust, SO16 6YD, UK

Peter Thom Clinical Genetics Service, Memorial Sloan-Kettering Cancer Center, New York, NY 10021, USA

Introduction

Boris Pasche

Cancer genetics is a rapidly evolving field, which has revolutionized the practice of medicine in the past decade. Genetic testing for several high-penetrance tumor susceptibility genes such as *BRCA1*, *BRCA2*, and *APC* have allowed the identification of individuals at high risk for breast and colon cancers that can be effectively prevented with early screening.

Somatically acquired genetic changes such as overexpression of the *ERBB2* gene in breast cancer and mutations of the *KRAS* or *BRAF* genes in colorectal cancer are observed in a significant fraction of patients. These genetic alterations can be effectively targeted with antibodies such as trastuzumab and cetuximab. Treatment with these genetically targeted agents increases patient survival.

Because genetic information allows for the exact identification of individuals, the widespread expansion of genetic testing is potentially fraught with ethical and legal issues. The first chapter of this book, which is written by Drs. Offit and Thom, provides an insightful overview of the ethical aspects of cancer genetics.

Systematic studies of common genetic variants are facilitated by the fact that individuals who carry a particular SNP allele at one site often predictably carry specific alleles at other nearby sites. This correlation is known as linkage disequilibrium (LD); a particular combination of alleles along a chromosome is termed a haplotype. The correlations between causal mutations and the haplotypes on which they arose have long served as a tool for human genetic research: first finding an association to a haplotype and then subsequently identifying the causal mutation(s) that it carries. With the sequencing of the human genome and development of high-throughput genomic methods, it has become clear that the human genome generally displays more LD than under simple population genetic models, and that LD is more varied across regions, and more segmentally structured, than had previously been supposed. These observations indicated that LD-based methods would generally have a great value (because nearby SNPs were typically correlated with many of the neighbors), and also that LD relationships would need to be empirically determined across

B. Pasche (✉)
Division of Hematology/Oncology, Department of Medicine, UAB Comprehensive Cancer Center, The University of Alabama, Birmingham, AL 35294-3300, USA
e-mail: boris.pasche@ccc.uab.edu

the genome by studying polymorphisms at high density in population samples. This has provided the rationale for the development of the International HapMap project (www.hapmap.org). Novel genotyping technologies combined with the knowledge generated by the HapMap project have provided the necessary tools to interrogate the association of genetic variants from the entire genome with risk for various diseases. The influence of such common polymorphisms on breast cancer, one of the leading causes of cancer death, is thoroughly reviewed in the second chapter written by Drs. Eccles and Tapper.

In the third chapter, Drs. Schrader and Huntsman provide the latest genetic knowledge related to gastric cancer and focus on genetic cause, identification, and management of a rare but deadly syndrome, hereditary gastric cancer.

Recent advances in cancer genetics are not limited to adult tumors. In the fourth chapter, Drs. Capasso and Diskin provide a timely update on the recent and exciting genetic discoveries related to one of the most common pediatric cancer, neuroblastoma.

In the fifth and last chapter, Drs. Bellam and Pasche review the latest discoveries related to constitutively altered TGF-β signaling in colorectal cancer risk, a novel phenotype that may account for a large proportion of colorectal cancers.

Chapter 1
Ethicolegal Aspects of Cancer Genetics

Kenneth Offit and Peter Thom

Abstract In the wake of efficacious preventive interventions based on hereditary cancer risk assessment, a number of ethical and legal challenges have emerged. These include issues such as appropriate testing of children and embryos, the "duty to warn" relatives about familial risk, reproductive genetic testing, the risk of genetic discrimination, and equitable access to testing. These and other issues will be discussed within the framework of a bioethical model, with reference to recent case law.

1 Introduction

While genetic information is clearly medical information, its uses and abuses may reach beyond the patient to the family and society. For these and other reasons, predictive genetic information, including the counseling that accompanies presymptomatic genetic testing, was introduced into the practice of clinical oncology as a special case requiring special considerations [1, 2]. At the time of the first widespread introduction of genetic testing for adult-onset breast, ovarian, and colon cancer, "genetic exceptionalism" was felt to be required because of the unique psychological, social, economic, and even political consequences of genetic information. Now, more than a decade later, it can be argued that genetic exceptionalism is no longer necessary. Moreover, the similarities between genetic and nongenetic predictive testing appear much greater than the differences [3]. In this review, the distinguishing characteristics and special ethical and legal implications of predictive genetic tests for cancer risk will be considered. The conclusion which will emerge is that breaking down genetic exceptionalism remains an important goal. However, achieving this goal will require continued physician and provider education and

K. Offit (✉)
Clinical Genetics Service, Memorial Sloan-Kettering Cancer Center, New York, NY 10021, USA
e-mail: offitk@mskcc.org

B. Pasche (ed.), *Cancer Genetics*, Cancer Treatment and Research 155,
DOI 10.1007/978-1-4419-6033-7_1, © Springer Science+Business Media, LLC 2010

also greater societal involvement in shaping the ethical discussions and case law that will determine the way genetic tests for cancer risk are being incorporated into the practice of preventive oncology.

2 Moral Theory: The Grounding of Biomedical Ethics

The moral implications of medical decisions and the use of newly introduced technologies have been examined by biomedical ethicists, and professional societies have entered into this dialogue by formulating uniform "codes" of professional ethics. Recent codes, including those of the AMA and the Office for Human Research Protections (OHRP), reflect the influence of modern ethical theory in the area of human genetic information [4, 5]. OHRP recommendations have become a critical resource for institutional IRBs and constitute basic reading for cancer risk counselors. Other professional organizations and advisory bodies have provided guidelines that bear on ethical and legal aspects of cancer genetic testing [1, 2, 6–8]. However, on many important issues (e.g., the duty to warn family members at risk and reproductive uses of genetic tests), clinicians and IRBs are expected to reach decisions based on the fundamental tenets of biomedical ethics. In the clinical setting, principle-driven normative ethics grounded in moral theory can guide individual ethical quandaries and have been specifically applied to cancer genetic testing [9].

In their classic introduction to biomedical ethics, Beauchamp and Childress [10] define the principles central to the current view of ethical conduct in medicine. These concepts include respect for individual autonomy of the patient; the imperative to do no harm (nonmaleficence); the concept of beneficence and justice; and specific obligations of the health professional relating to truth telling, privacy, confidentiality, and morally correct behavior.

3 Autonomy

The principle of autonomy is perhaps the most fundamental to genetic medicine. Strictly defined, autonomy refers to self-rule, but in bioethical parlance this concept is more broadly defined. It refers to the right of the individual to act freely, when provided adequate information, without coercion or interference. The concept of autonomy has also been invoked to justify the individual's right not to know medical information. Cancer genetic counseling, with its emphasis on education and empowerment, is fully consistent with the concept of autonomy, implying fully informed choice, free from coercion. The context of testing presumptively nonautonomous children and embryos raises special concerns, which will be discussed below.

4 Nonmaleficence

The Hippocratic maxim primum non nocere – "above all do no harm" – has become a central dogma in medical ethics. Nonmaleficence, as it relates to cancer patients, has major application to genetic testing. False-negative tests may be avoided by establishing segregation of a pathogenic mutation by initiating testing of an affected family member. However, for common malignancies such as colon or breast cancer, where significant population risk exists, even a "true negative genetic test may be deleterious if the individual abandons cancer screening." Negative test results may also, paradoxically, result in "survivor guilt." The damaging effects of positive test results appear self-evident. For some conditions, such as Li–Fraumeni syndrome, the harm:benefit ratio of testing may be a central consideration. For those circumstances where a genetic test will lead to increased surveillance or risk-reducing surgery, there can be medical risks to these procedures. However, the greatest perceived risk associated with genetic testing has been a nonmedical one: the troubling adverse psychological, social, and economic consequences of stigmatization and genetic discrimination against mutation carriers.

5 Genetic Discrimination

Genetic discrimination is defined as social stigmatization based on an individual's hereditary risk of disease. It can lead to purely social traumas, such as discrimination against potential spouses due entirely to their disease risk. Genetic discrimination can create economic hardship, for example, when genetic knowledge is used by potential employers in hiring or promotion decisions or by insurance carriers to exclude groups from coverage or to increase their rates. While anecdotally documented for a number of rarer disorders, this concern has been mainly theoretical for common adult cancer predisposition syndromes, with very few documented cases of insurance discrimination thus far [11, 12]. Nonetheless, the perceived fear of genetic discrimination remains high [13]. Early surveys of medical directors of US life insurance companies found that more than half felt a strong family history of breast cancer justified them to disallow all life insurance or substantially increase rates [14]. In some countries, e.g., the UK, life insurance premiums are higher for those with *BRCA* mutations. From the perspective of "distributive justice," combined with the notion of life insurance as a commodity and not a right, the option of excluding high-risk groups to guarantee the lowest possible rates seems logical. Antiselection, the bane of insurers, occurs when those at increased risk more actively seek insurance. Health insurance, on the other hand, tends to be viewed more as a right than a commodity, hence the ethical arguments against genetic discrimination in the workplace, the context in which most health insurance is provided in the USA.

5.1 Federal and State Legislation and Case Law

Several cases involving genetic discrimination in the workplace have been reported. In *Norman-Bloodsaw v. Lawrence Berkeley Laboratory* [15] the courts decided in favor of the plaintiffs who were subjected to preemployment genetic screening at Lawrence Berkeley Laboratory. The plaintiffs alleged that their blood and urine samples were tested for a variety of conditions including sickle cell trait without prior knowledge, consent, or subsequent notification that the tests had been conducted. In theory, the Americans with Disabilities Act [16] prevents employers from inquiring about health conditions in the course of evaluation for employment. This protection was further strengthened when the Equal Employment Opportunity Commission (EEOC) [17] promulgated enforcement guidelines, March 15, 1995, defining "disability" as inclusive of genetic predisposition. In a far-reaching case that tested the scope of the EEOC regulation, Burlington Northern Santa Fe Railway Company conducted genetic tests on blood samples of employees who had filed workers' compensation claims for carpal tunnel syndrome. Under the terms of a settlement in *EEOC v. Burlington N. Santa Fe Ry. Co.* [No.02-C-0456 (E.D. Wis. 2002)], the company agreed to stop the testing.

In addition to the EEOC provisions, several other federal initiatives impact upon the potential for discrimination by health insurers or employers based on genetic knowledge. The Health Insurance Portability and Accountability Act (HIPAA) defined genetic information as a component of the "health status" of the individual, along with obvious manifestations of disease, disability, and medical history. The intent of the legislation was to prohibit both employers and health insurers from excluding individuals, or employees in a group, from coverage or from charging them higher rates on the basis of health status, including genetic conditions. The legislation's intent was also to spread risk among insurance pools, while protecting individuals with specific conditions from losing the portability of their insurance when they changed jobs. Hence, for cancer patients in clinics who undergo genetic testing, federal protection was put in place to shield them from discrimination based on genetic test results. Other provisions of HIPAA laid down strict rules governing privacy of protected health information. However, no provisions for recourse were established when privacy has been violated and over 16,000 privacy violation complaints have been filed to HHS since the enactment of HIPAA privacy rules in 1996 [18]. In 2006, during testimony before the United States Senate HELP Committee, 35% of Fortune 500 companies admitted to looking at an employee's health records before hiring and promotion decisions were made [19]. As the USA moves to implement a digitized medical record system, balancing privacy issues against the benefits of ready access to patients' electronic records will remain an important issue.

In 2000, President Bill Clinton signed an executive order prohibiting discrimination in federal employment based on genetic information [20]. Under the leadership of the Senate Majority Leader who was also a physician, a bipartisan effort resulted in the unanimous passage of the Genetic Information Nondiscrimination Act, S. 306. on February 17, 2005, by a 98–0 margin. More than 3 years later the House of Representatives version of the legislation, H.R. 493, was passed. The Genetic Information Nondiscrimination Act (GINA) of 2008, signed into law by President George W. Bush, prohibits discrimination based on genetic information in health coverage and employment. GINA also provides remedies for violations, including corrective action and monetary penalties. Individuals may also have the right to pursue private litigation [21].

The HIPAA and GINA protections were meant to provide baseline protections against genetic discrimination; they are subordinate to state regulations with more stringent genetic confidentiality and protection guidelines. By 2007, the majority of states had passed various types of legislation bearing on issues of genetic discrimination. Genetic privacy statutes have been passed by 32 states. In 27 states there are specific consent provisions for disclosure of genetic information. The provisions of the state laws with respect to health insurance vary, but generally parallel the legislation on privacy and employer discrimination. A comprehensive, constantly updated source for state laws governing genetics and privacy issues can be found at the Web site for the National Conference of State Legislatures (http://www.ncsl.org). The impact of many of these state laws is limited by the Employee Retirement Income Security Act (ERISA), which preempts self-insured employers from many of the state insurance provisions. From the perspective of the individual with a genetic predisposition to cancer, one of the potential benefits of the Health Insurance Portability and Accountability laws is that they apply to employers providing health insurance plans, including small employers (with 2–50 employees).

Consumers' perceptions that genetic testing may lead to discrimination are well established by surveys and polls, regardless of actual occurrence [22, 23]. In actual practice, major health insurers have included cancer genetic testing as a covered benefit. Some carriers, like Aetna and Blue Cross, cover cancer genetic testing and do not explicitly require test results to be sent to their databases. Insurance carriers have also covered the cost for risk-reducing surgeries associated with cancer predisposition syndromes; in our series greater than 95% of preventive surgeries of the breast or ovaries were covered [24]. In addition, case law has supported this practice; in a 1994 case, an asymptomatic woman, whose mother and aunt had both died of ovarian cancer in their late forties, elected to have a total abdominal hysterectomy and bilateral salpingo-oophorectomy. The Nebraska Supreme Court reversed an earlier decision supporting BlueCross/Blue shield, which had refused payment for the procedure. In this case the woman had not had confirmatory genetic testing, but the courts upheld her contention that though there was no detectable physical evidence of illness she did "suffer from a different or abnormal genetic constitution." [25]

5.2 Direct-to-Consumer(DTC) Genetic Testing

One of the potential harms of genetic testing is psychological damage resulting from poor or absent genetic counseling. Inaccurate performance or interpretation of genetic testing may also lead to inappropriate clinical decisions. Both of these concerns have re-emerged in the context of discussions of direct-to-consumer (DTC) marketing of genetic tests.

Arguments for DTC testing hinge on greater access to information. Arguments against DTC testing are that consumers may not be educated to understand the complexities of genetic testing, may misinterpret results, and may consequently make health management errors. Concerns about consumer education were supported by an "experiment" that took place in Atlanta, GA, and Denver, CO, during September 2002–February 2003. A large genetic testing company embarked on a DTC advertising campaign for *BRCA* testing. At the same time the Centers for Disease Control studied several comparison cities: Raleigh and Durham, NC, and Seattle, WA. Television and media advertisements were highly effective, reaching 90% of the homes in the selected markets. It was noted that consumer and provider awareness of *BRCA1/2* testing increased, more *BRCA1/2* tests were requested, and more tests ordered. In all four cities, health-care providers often lacked sufficient knowledge to advise patients about genetic testing. In Denver, there was a 300% increase in calls from women interested in *BRCA* testing, but a 30% decrease in referral of high-risk women during the campaign. It was concluded that advertising campaign may not have accurately portrayed the limitations of *BRCA* testing [26].

In addition there is considerable controversy concerning the analytical and clinical validity of some tests currently offered [27]. DTC laboratories' inclusion of risk markers identified through genome-wide association studies has presented new challenges: the predictive value of most of these markers remains theoretical and in many instances their genetic function is unknown. Quality control standards are not yet in place for physician-directed genetic testing. Basic requirements exist under the Clinical Laboratory Improvement Amendments of 1988 (CLIA), but there are no specific mandates covering proficiency testing of personnel, or quality control of genetics labs, though many do voluntarily comply with industry-set standards. In 2000, the Secretary's Advisory Committee on Genetic Testing (SACGT) issued a report proposing that genetic testing be regulated under CLIA and that new genetic tests should be reviewed by the FDA. A recent analysis of the number of reported deficiencies and the frequency of reported analytic errors has shown that proficiency testing of laboratory technicians is clearly associated with better laboratory quality [28].

Regulation of laboratories involved in DTC genetic testing falls under the purview of individual states, and uniformity is lacking: Some prohibit delivery of test results directly to patients, some do not, and still others have no governing statutes covering this issue. There also appears to be a wide range in quality of direct-to-consumer testing facilities. One online company offers testing for *BRCA* carrier status. Full sequencing is listed at over $3,000 and includes "expert support by board-certified genetics experts, toll-free or via email." Another company offers a range of both established and poorly established genomic markers that allegedly predict possible health proclivities and even include dietary modifications based on genotype. Some of these DTC tests are coupled with the sale of products claiming to treat the ailments identified by the tests or to "match" one's genetic profile, such as "customized" supplements to aid in weight loss [29]. While the Federal Trade Commission has exercised authority over prescription drug advertising, it has not yet regulated the arena of DTC genetic testing.

6 Beneficence

One of the fundamental benefits of genetic counseling is the psychological benefit of a "negative" test, but a "positive" genetic test can also be considered beneficent if it leads to more effective medical management. While early studies recognized the presumed but unproven efficacy of such interventions as mammography, breast self-examination, ovarian screening, colonoscopy, and prophylactic surgery in carriers of cancer predisposing alleles [30], more recent literature [31, 32] has supported the efficacy of these interventions for a broad spectrum of adult and pediatric cancer predisposition syndromes. "Preventive" ovarian surgery in *BRCA* mutation carriers, for example, results in the detection of microscopic and curable ovarian cancer in 3 of every 100 women who undergo the procedure [33], and colonoscopies can detect small tumors at a curable stage [34].

7 Paternalism: The Collision of Beneficence and Autonomy

In some cases, the principles of autonomy and beneficence collide. When, for example, the perceived necessity to inform a patient's relatives clashes with the right of that patient not to disclose medical information, the medical provider's choice to disclose information to family members may appear paternalistic. Such dilemmas have resulted in an established set of case law referred to as "duty to warn" implying a possible ethical obligation for the practitioner to invoke beneficent considerations and indeed, in some circumstances, to override the autonomy of the proband by informing at-risk relatives [35]. In several examples of recent case law, legal claims have been made against physicians for failing to warn relatives of hereditary cancer risks. In one case of hereditary medullary thyroid cancer in Florida, *Pate v. Threlkel* [661 So.2d 278 (Fla. 1995)], the court ruled that warning the affected proband was sufficient familial notification. Expanding on this opinion in another case involving familial polyposis, *Safer v. Pack* [677 A. 2d 1188 (N.J. 1996)], the New Jersey Superior Court did not agree that "in all circumstances the duty to warn will be satisfied by informing the patient." This case and a third case involving a noncancerous condition may establish a precedent in other states and create special challenges in the counseling and testing of families with hereditary cancer predisposition [36].

Under HIPAA there are specific "public interest" exceptions to the strict nondisclosure policy that otherwise protects "individually identifiable health information," including genetic information. These exceptions comprise instances in which the public interest is at risk, i.e., there is a "serious and imminent threat to the health or safety of a person or the public" [37]; and the physician has the capacity to avert significant harm [38]. At present ASCO and AMA guidelines state that the clinician is obligated to inform the proband of the familial risks that must be communicated to relatives, but that it is impractical and inappropriate to create liabilities for clinicians to warn all relatives of possible genetic risk for a malignancy [35]. Setting aside the issue of duty to warn the family of genetic risk, there is little debate about the duty to warn the individual patient. Already there has been a malpractice suit settled for $1.6 million against a prominent Seattle, Washington, medical center not only for failure to make a genetic diagnosis in a patient with a family history of breast and ovarian cancer but in neglecting to offer risk-reducing ovarian surgery to a 43-year-old woman who survived bilateral breast cancer at ages 28 and 37 only to succumb to ovarian cancer at age 43 [39]. Such cases underscore the importance of oncologists' abilities to identify their patients' hereditary cancer syndromes in light of estimates that 5–10% of the 2.5 million existing survivors of breast and colon cancer in the USA are at risk for a second cancer due to an underlying, often unrecognized, hereditary cancer syndrome.

8 Veracity

The concern with truth telling is a relatively recent one in biomedical ethics [10]. In virtually every case involving cancer genetics, the rules of disclosure should be anticipated during the pretest counseling. A special consideration, and a potentially devastating disclosure unique to genetic testing, is the issue of relatedness (i.e., paternity and maternity). Since cancer predisposition testing is generally performed on families with adult members, the issue of non-relatedness among family members generally arises unexpectedly, and the resulting emotional and legal consequences may be significant. The preferred solution to these particular dilemmas of veracity is to proactively anticipate the problem during the pretest stage and to establish whether this information is to be disclosed or is deemed irrelevant to the immediate medical concerns.

9 Equity

Although not usually considered in the context of genetic testing of individuals, ethical consideration of equity and access is relevant to the responsible translation of molecular medicine.

European studies have described an overrepresentation of upper-class women and the corresponding deficit among lower-class women with breast cancer who were referred to genetics clinics [40]. Acceptance of *BRCA*1/2 test results is also limited in US African American women [41], and although expectations among

African Americans about the benefits of *BRCA*1/2 genetic testing were high, exposure to information and knowledge about breast cancer genetics was lacking [42]. Factors contributing to or preventing participation in genetic testing among African Americans may include awareness of epidemiological data showing lower survival rates among African American cancer patients, leading to fatalistic attitudes. In these studies, education and income were important determinants of attitudes, beliefs, and behaviors, and larger studies have shown African American participants were significantly less likely to have had genetic counseling (OR 0.22; 95% CI, 0.12–0.40). After controlling for probability of carrying a mutation, socioeconomic factors, cancer risk perceptions and worry, attitudes about the risks and benefits of testing, and primary care physician discussions about testing, a significant odds ratio persisted (0.28; 95% CI, 0.09–0.89). Though access to health care in the USA is nominally linked to employment status, fully 67% of uninsured individuals were in families where at least one person worked full time during 2005 [43]. And during the same year, nearly two of three (62%) Hispanics were uninsured at some point compared to 33% of African Americans and 20% of European Americans [44]. Thus, barriers to mammograms, colonoscopies, and genetic testing, as well as cancer treatment, are formidable, and for the working poor this cost barrier may contribute to later-stage diagnoses and late treatment for cancer.

10 Special Considerations: Genetic Testing of Children and Fetuses

Current AMA guidelines for genetic testing of children attempt to strike a balance between preserving the child's autonomy versus considerations about imminence of risk to the child or relative and availability of therapeutic measures. Carrier testing children for a late-onset genetic condition is not recommended, whereas genetic testing for an early-onset disease with available treatment options is recommended and sometimes required. When no treatment is available for children at risk for an early-onset disease, the AMA suggests the option to test the child be placed at parents' discretion [45]. When the balance of harms and benefits is uncertain some professional guidelines, such as those of the ACMG, are somewhat more open to testing children. These guidelines do consider psychosocial benefits which may warrant offering tests to competent adolescents [46]. ASCO recommends that the decision to offer testing to potentially affected children should consider the availability of evidence-based risk-reduction strategies and the probability that malignancy will develop during childhood. The National Association of Genetic Counselors (NSGC) goes still further in advocating offering prenatal testing for adult-onset genetic conditions without regard to decisions about terminating an affected fetus [47]. While some have proposed that parental authority is an important consideration that may outweigh hypothetical harm and that decisions to test should be case specific [48], others have challenged the notion that maturity of judgment is universally age related [49].

11 Embryonic Genetic Testing

At the far end of this spectrum lies the issue of genetic testing where definitions of personhood and the autonomy are unclarified. Techniques used to identify the presence of disease-associated genes in a fetus include traditional postimplantation methods, amniocentesis and CVS, and preimplantation genetic diagnosis (PGD). Use of PGD in IVF affords the option of embryonic selection through detection of single-gene or chromosomal disorders at a very early stage of embryonic life. We reviewed the peer-reviewed literature and found 55 case reports of prenatal or preimplantation diagnoses for cancer predisposition syndromes [50]. We found that 9 of 13 PGD centers contacted indicated that they already offered or planned to offer such services. Professional societies are active participants in discussing the regulation of PGD and other assisted reproductive technologies. Although the American Medical Association's (AMA's) Code of Medical Ethics finds it generally acceptable to use prenatal genetic testing for individuals at "elevated risk of fetal genetic disorders," the AMA states that "selection to avoid a genetic disease may not always be appropriate, depending on factors such as the severity of the disease, the probability of its occurrence, the age at onset, and the time of gestation at which selection would occur" [51]; comparable positions have been taken by the ethics committee of the American Society of Reproductive Medicine [52] and by various European medical ethics societies [53–55].

Ethical concerns arise in the context of PGD because some feel that offering a routine option of termination for late-onset diseases risks the "slippery slope" leading to sex and trait selection or testing for multifactorial conditions, such as depression or obesity. In addition, with increased uptake, the ethical issue of equal access arises because currently this technology is affordable only by a select few. In the absence of data on long-term outcome for assisted reproductive technologies [56], and absent guidelines for practitioners to discuss such options with patients, an algorithm to approach these discussions – taking into account psychological, ethical, as well as medical considerations – has been proposed [57].

12 Informed Consent and the Unifying Concept of Fidelity

In the absence of the contractual obligations of the marketplace, the concept of fidelity has been invoked to capture the spirit of trust, commitment, and faithfulness that exists in the doctor–patient relationship. Arising from the necessity to make explicit the agreement between patient and health provider, especially in the face of difficult decisions, and in keeping with the principles of autonomous choice, the concept of informed consent was developed. The basic requirements of informed consent are (1) competence to understand the informed consent discussion; (2) disclosure of procedures, risks, and benefits of the research; (3) understanding of what has been discussed; (4) voluntariness of the decision; and (5) consent by the individual or the appropriate surrogate. For the most part, pretest genetic counseling is synonymous with informed consent. Table 1.1 lists the basic elements of informed consent for genetic cancer predisposition testing, grouped according to the aspect of ethical theory that they address.

Table 1.1 Elements of informed consent for germline cancer risk testing

Autonomy provisions

1. Information about the specific test being performed
2. Implications of both positive and negative results
3. Possibility that the test will be inconclusive or not informative
4. Options for estimating risk without genetic testing
5. Risk for children to inherit the mutation
6. Options to withdraw from study

Beneficence provisions

7. Options for medical surveillance, risk reduction, and screening following testing

Nonmaleficence provisions

8. Technical accuracy of testing
9. Risks of psychological distress
10. Risks of insurance and/or employer discrimination

Paternalism provisions

11. Procedures if relatedness is unexpected
12. Procedures for notification of family

Privacy-professional responsibilities

13. Confidentiality issues
14. Fees for testing, counseling, and follow-up care

Special considerations

15. Ownership and research uses of DNA remaining after diagnostic testing
16. Reproductive uses of genetic information

References

1. American Society of Clinical Oncology (1996) Statement of the American Society of Clinical Oncology: genetic testing for cancer susceptibility. J Clin Oncol 14:1730–1736
2. American Society of Clinical Oncology (2003) American Society of Clinical Oncology policy statement update: genetic testing for cancer susceptibility. J Clin Oncol 21:2397–2406
3. Green MJ, Botkin JR (2003) "Genetic exceptionalism" in medicine: clarifying the differences between genetic and nongenetic tests. Ann Intern Med 138:571–575
4. American Medical Association Opinions on social policy issues, 1/4/05 update. http://www.ama-assn.org/ama/pub/category/8295.html. Accessed 1/5/2007
5. United States Department of Health and Human Services Office for human research protection (OHRP) policy guidance [by topics], 12/28/06 update. http://www.hhs.gov/ohrp/policy/index.html. Accessed 5/07/09

6. The National Women's Health Information Center (1996) Position paper: hereditary susceptibility testing for breast cancer, March 1996, 5/7/02 update. http://www.4woman.gov/napbc/catalog.wci/napbc/hspospap.htm. Accessed 1/5/07
7. National Information Resource on Ethics and Human Genetics 3/06 update. http://bioethics.georgetown.edu/nirehg/. Accessed 4/18/09
8. Genetics & Public Policy Center http://www.dnapolicy.org/. Accessed 5/07/09
9. Offit K (1998) Chapter 10. In: Clinical cancer genetics: risk management and counseling. Wiley, New York
10. Beauchamp TL, Childress JF (1994) Principles of biomedical ethics. Oxford University Press, New York
11. Hall MA, Rich SS (2000) Laws restricting health insurers' use of genetic information: impact on genetic discrimination. Am J Hum Genet 66:293–307
12. Harris M, Winship I, Spriggs M (2005) Controversies and ethical issues in cancer-genetics clinics. Lancet Oncol 6:301–310
13. Hall MA, McEwen JE, Barton JC et al (2005) Concerns in a primary care population about genetic discrimination by insurers. Genet Med 7:311–316
14. McEwen JE, McCarty K, Reilly PR (1992) A survey of state insurance commissioners concerning genetic testing and life insurance. Am J Hum Genet 51:785–792
15. Norman-Bloodsaw v. Lawrence Berkeley Laboratory 135 F.3d 1260, 1269 (9th Cir. 1998)
16. The U.S. Equal Employment Opportunity Commission (EEOC) The Americans with disabilities act of 1990, Title I and V. US Code 12111–12201. http://www.eeoc.gov/policy/ada.html. Accessed 5/07/09
17. The U.S. Equal Employment Opportunity Commission (EEOC) Compliance manual, vol. 2, section 902, order 9 15.002, 902–945, 6/06 update. http://www.eeoc.gov/policy/ada.html. Accessed 5/07/09
18. Patient Privacy Rights. http://www.patientprivacyrights.org/site/PageServer. Accessed 5/07/09
19. 65 Fed. Reg. 82,467
20. Clinton WJ (2000) Executive Order 13145 of February 8, 2000: to prohibit discrimination in federal employment based on genetic information. Fed Regist 65:6877–6880
21. Genetic Information Nondiscrimination Act (GINA) of 2008. Information for researchers and health care professionals. http://www.genome.gov/24519851. Accessed 4/18/09
22. Lapham EV, Kozma C, Weiss JO (1996) Genetic discrimination: perspectives of consumers. Science 274:621–624
23. Statement of Commissioner Paul Steven Miller, U.S. Equal Employment Opportunity Commission (20 July 2000). "Genetic information in the workplace." Before the Committee on Health, Education, Labor and Pensions, U.S. Senate
24. Kauff ND, Mitra N, Robson ME et al (2005) Risk of ovarian cancer in BRCA1 and BRCA2 mutation-negative hereditary breast cancer families. J Natl Cancer Inst 97:1382–1384
25. Katskee v. Blue Cross/Blue Shield. Nebraska (1994) 515 N.W.2d 645
26. Centers for Disease Control and Prevention (CDC) (2004) Genetic testing for breast and ovarian cancer susceptibility: evaluating direct-to-consumer marketing–Atlanta, Denver, Raleigh-Durham, and Seattle, 2003. MMWR 53:603–606
27. Hogarth S, Javitt G, Melzer D (2008) The current landscape for direct-to-consumer genetic testing: legal, ethical, and policy issues. Annu Rev Genomics Hum Genet 9:161–182
28. Hudson KL, Murphy JA, Kaufman DJ et al (2006) Oversight of US genetic testing laboratories. Nat Biotechnol 24:1083–1090
29. Hudson K (2006). Testimony before the United States senate special committee on aging "at home DNA tests: marketing scam or medical breakthrough?" 27 July 2006. http://www.dnapolicy.org/resources/Testimony_of_Kathy_Hudson_Senate_Aging_7-27-06.pdf. Accessed 12/01/2006
30. Burke W, Petersen G, Lynch P et al (1997) Recommendations for follow-up care of individuals with an inherited predisposition to cancer. I. Hereditary nonpolyposis colon cancer. Cancer Genetics Studies Consortium. JAMA 277:915–919; Burke W, Daly M, Garber J, et al (1997)

Recommendations for follow-up care of individuals with an inherited predisposition to cancer. II. BRCA1 and BRCA2. Cancer Genetics Studies Consortium. JAMA 277:997–1003

31. Offit K, Garber J, Grady M et al (2004) American society of clinical oncology curriculum: cancer genetics and cancer predisposition testing, 2nd edn. ASCO Publishing, Alexandria, VA

32. Robson M, Offit K (2007) Management of women at hereditary risk for breast cancer. N Engl J Med 357:154–162

33. Kauff ND, Satagopan JM, Robson ME et al (2002) Risk-reducing salpingo-oophorectomy in women with a BRCA1 or BRCA2 mutation. N Engl J Med 346:1609–1615

34. Garber J, Offit K (2005) Hereditary cancer predisposition syndromes. J Clin Oncol 23:276–292

35. Offit K, Groeger E, Turner S et al (2004) The "duty to warn" a patient's family members about hereditary disease risks. JAMA 292:1469–1473

36. Burke T, Rosenbaum S (2005) Molloy v Meier and the expanding standard of medical care: implications for public health policy and practice. Public Health Rep 120:209–210

37. Andrews LB (1994) Assessing genetic risks: implications for health and social policy. National Academy Press, Washington, DC

38. Reilly PR, Boshar MF, Holtzman SH (1997) Ethical issues in genetic research: disclosure and informed consent. Nat Genet 15:16–20

39. Miletich S, Armstrong K, Mayo J (2006) Life or death question, but debate was hidden for years. Seattle Times, 19 Oct 2006

40. Carstairs VDL, Morris R (1991) Deprivation and health in Scotland. Aberdeen. Aberdeen University Press, Aberdeen

41. Halbert CH, Kessler L, Stopfer JE et al (2006) Low rates of acceptance of BRCA1 and BRCA2 test results among African American women at increased risk for hereditary breast-ovarian cancer. Genet Med 8:576–582

42. Halbert CH, Kessler LJ, Mitchell E (2005) Genetic testing for inherited breast cancer risk in African Americans. Cancer Invest 23:285–295

43. Collins SR, Davis K, Doty MM et al (2006) Gaps in health insurance: an all-American problem: findings from the commonwealth fund biennial health insurance survey, April 2006. http://www.commonwealthfund.org/usr_doc/Collins_gapshltins_920.pdf. Accessed 4/29/09

44. Doty MM, Holmgren AL (2006) Health care disconnect: gaps in coverage and care for minority adults. Findings from the commonwealth fund biennial health insurance survey (2005). Issue Brief (Commonwealth Fund) 21:1–12

45. AMA Opinions on social policy issues, E-2.138, Genetic Testing of Children

46. American Society of Human Genetics Board of Directors, American College of Medical Genetics Board of Directors (1995) Points to consider: ethical, legal, and psychosocial implications of genetic testing in children and adolescents. Am J Hum Genet 57:1233–1241

47. National Society of Genetic Counselors Position Statement: Prenatal And Childhood Testing For Adult-Onset Disorders, adopted 2005. http://www.nsgc.org/about/position.cfm#Prenatal_two. Accessed 5/07/09

48. Rhodes R (2006) Why test children for adult-onset genetic diseases? Mt Sinai J Med 73:609–616

49. Cauffman E, Steinberg L (2000) (Im)maturity of judgment in adolescence: why adolescents may be less culpable than adults. Behav Sci Law 18:741–760

50. Offit K, Kohut K, Clagett B et al (2006) Cancer genetic testing and assisted reproduction. J Clin Oncol 24:1–8

51. The Council on Ethical and Judicial Affairs, American Medical Association (1994) Ethical issues related to prenatal genetic testing. Arch Fam Med 3:633–642

52. Ethics Committee of the American Society of Reproductive Medicine (2004) Sex selection and preimplantation genetic diagnosis. Fertil Steril 82:S245–S248

53. British Medical Association. Preimplantation genetic diagnosis with tissue typing, 10/99 update.http://www.bma.org.uk/ap.nsf/AttachmentsByTitle/PDFEthicsBrief68/$FILE/EthicsBrief68.pdf. Accessed 12/03/06

54. Thornhill AR, de Die-Smulders CE, Geraedts JP et al (2005) ESHRE PGD consortium 'best practice guidelines for clinical preimplantation genetic diagnosis (PGD) and preimplantation genetic screening (PGS)'. Hum Reprod 20:35–48
55. Danish Council of Ethics. Microinsemination and pre-implantation genetic diagnosis (PGD): resume of recommendations, 3/05 update. http://www.etiskraad.dk/sw1771.asp. Accessed 5/07/09
56. The President's Council on Bioethics. Reproduction and responsibility: the regulation of new biotechnologies, 3/04 update. Accessed 12/03/06
57. Offit K, Sagi M, Hurley K (2006) Preimplantation genetic diagnosis for cancer syndromes: a new challenge for preventive medicine. JAMA 296:2727–2730

Chapter 2
The Influence of Common Polymorphisms on Breast Cancer

Diana Eccles and William Tapper

Abstract Breast cancer is one of the most frequently diagnosed cancers in the Western world and a significant cause of mortality worldwide. A small proportion of cases are accounted for by high-penetrance monogenic predisposition genes; however, this explains only a small fraction (less than 5%) of all breast cancers. Increasingly with advances in molecular technology and the development of large research consortia, the locations and identities of many low-penetrance genetic variants are being discovered. However, each variant has a very small effect similar to or smaller than many of the known environmental risk factors. It is therefore unlikely that these variants will be appropriate for predictive genetic testing, although they may identify novel pathways and genes which provide new insights and targets for therapeutic intervention. The future challenges will be identifying causal variants and determining how these low-penetrance alleles interact with each other and with environmental factors in order to usefully implement them in the practice of clinical medicine. Furthermore, it is clear that breast cancer comes in many forms with the tumour pathology and immunohistochemical profile already being used routinely as prognostic indicators and to inform treatment decisions. However, these indicators of prognosis are imperfect; two apparently identical tumours may have very different outcomes in different individuals. Inherited genetic variants may well be one of the other factors that need to be taken into account in assessing prognosis and planning treatment.

1 Introduction

Like most common cancers there is good evidence from population, family, and twin studies that shared genetic variants are contributing a proportion of risk [1, 2].

D. Eccles (✉)
Human Genetics and Cancer Sciences Divisions, School of Medicine, University of Southampton, Southampton University Hospitals NHS Trust, SO16 6YD, UK
e-mail: d.m.eccles@soton.ac.uk

B. Pasche (ed.), *Cancer Genetics*, Cancer Treatment and Research 155,
DOI 10.1007/978-1-4419-6033-7_2, © Springer Science+Business Media, LLC 2010

Close relatives of an individual with breast cancer have an increased risk of developing the disease. In some (relatively rare) families there is a striking, dominant pattern of breast cancer, often in association with ovarian cancer. In these families, a likely explanation is a dominantly inherited rare genetic variant (mutation) with a high lifetime penetrance for breast (and ovarian) cancer. The two most frequently mutated high-penetrance breast cancer genes are *BRCA1* and *BRCA2* [3]. The chance of breast cancer in a family being due to a single dominantly inherited gene increases with an increasing number of affected relatives; young age at onset and multiple primary tumours in an individual are characteristic of genetic predisposition, and these features are often used to select individuals for genetic counselling and genetic testing to determine if there is a high-risk gene mutation present in the family [4]. The lifetime age-related penetrance in a family that was ascertained because of multiple affected family members can be as high as 80% by 70 years of age [5]. However, it is clear that the penetrance of these high-risk genes varies between individuals and between families. At least some of this variation is associated with the presence of common genetic polymorphisms [6]. In many families with clustering of breast cancer, the pattern is less striking than in families with a *BRCA1* or *BRCA2* mutation. Figure 2.1 illustrates a pattern of inheritance in a family that is likely to have arisen because of a *BRCA1* gene mutation. Figure 2.2 is a family unlikely to have arisen as a result of a *BRCA1* or *BRCA2* mutation but also unlikely to have occurred entirely by coincidence; this familial cluster of breast cancers is most likely to have arisen because of a combination of shared low-penetrance genes and environmental factors.

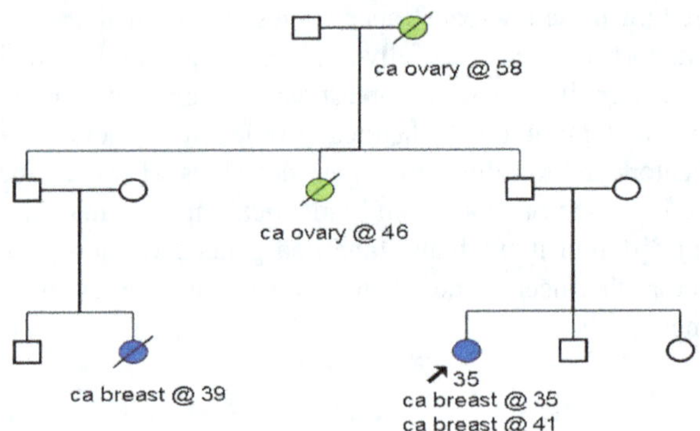

Fig. 2.1 Family history likely to be due to a *BRCA1* gene mutation

2 Breast Cancer Epidemiology

Breast cancer is one of the commonest cancers in the Western world and the incidence has been increasing over the last 25 years particularly in the more frequently affected post-menopausal age groups (http://info.cancerresearchuk.org/cancerstats/types/breast/). The strongest risk factors for breast cancer are sex (male breast cancer

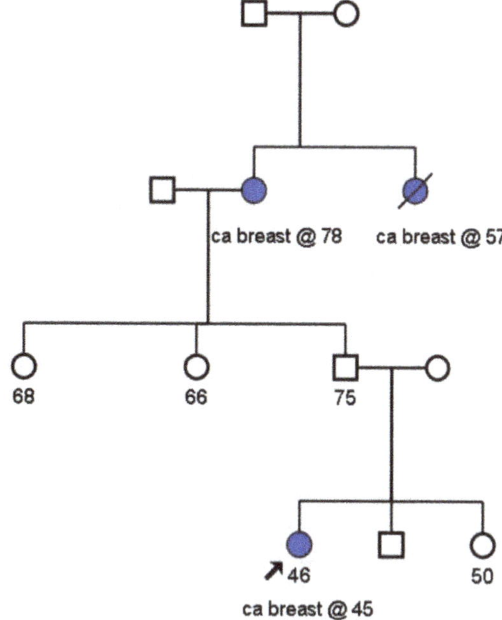

Fig. 2.2 Family history is likely due to low-penetrance breast cancer risk alleles BRCA1 gene mutation

incidence is much lower than for females) and age (in the UK and USA 80% of all breast cancers are diagnosed in women over 50 years of age). Obesity, early age at menarche, late age at menopause, late age at first birth, use of hormone replacement therapy after menopause, current use of oral contraceptive pills, sedentary lifestyle, and alcohol consumption are all factors that have been reported to impact on breast cancer risk. Some of these factors are entirely environmental (e.g. oral contraceptive pill use) and some such as obesity are a combination of complex genetic traits, lifestyle, and environment. Changes in lifestyle can exert an effect on breast cancer risk over a relatively short time scale [7, 8].

3 Breast Cancer Biology

Breast cancer is clearly both pathologically and molecularly more than one disease [9]. Routine pathological examination can and is used to subdivide tumour types since these give information about the likely prognosis and the need for additional treatment (surgery, hormonal manipulation, cytotoxic, or targeted drugs) [10, 11]. In addition to studying the morphological features of a breast tumour, the tissue will be examined using immunohistochemistry to determine, for example, whether a tumour has oestrogen receptors (ER positive) or not (ER negative). Most breast cancers (80%) express oestrogen receptors (are ER positive) and are therefore likely to respond to anti-oestrogen treatments. More recently amplification of a transmembrane tyrosine kinase epidermal growth factor receptor HER2 has been clearly associated with a poor prognosis. Only a small proportion of breast cancers (<20%) show overexpression of HER2 but the recent development of therapeutic antibodies targeted at HER2 has rapidly established a need to identify those patients who might benefit from this targeted therapy [9, 12].

Increasingly sophisticated molecular techniques are now being used to analyse RNA and DNA extracted from tumours and identify several different molecular subgroups of breast cancer that are associated with differing clinical outcomes [13–15]. Despite this increasing sophistication of analysis of tumour types and the broad association of patterns of pathological or molecular features with overall prognosis, it is still not possible to precisely predict for any single individual when or where they will relapse from a tumour with any measure of certainty.

Black African women are known to develop breast cancer at a younger average age than white Caucasian populations and for breast tumours to be more likely to have adverse prognostic characteristics, specifically more oestrogen receptor negative tumours [16, 17]. This could be due to different genetic backgrounds and the presence of more low-penetrance risk alleles predisposing to ER-negative rather than ER-positive breast cancers in association with Black African ancestry. Breast cancer in younger women relative to post-menopausal women typically involves a higher prevalence of tumour types with adverse pathological features [18, 19]. This may be due to a difference in either the host environment, causative factors (genetic and environmental), or both. Female *BRCA1* gene mutation carriers are much more likely than most women to be affected with breast cancer at young ages but even in comparison to young women without *BRCA1* mutations, the likelihood of an ER-negative breast cancer developing in a *BRCA1* gene mutation carrier is extremely high [20]. This suggests that the high-risk gene mutation may be facilitating a particular molecular pathway of tumour evolution.

4 Breast Cancer Diagnosis

The diagnosis of breast cancer may be based on clinical examination and radiological features but a definitive diagnosis requires a pathological assessment of tumour tissue. This gives information about the growth rate of tumour cells (tumour nuclear grade is made up of a combined score where the pathologist assesses tubule formation, nuclear pleomorphism, and mitotic count), the type of breast cancer (e.g. ductal or lobular or one of the special subtypes), and with specific antibody stains the immunohistochemical profile (usually at least ER and HER2 receptor status). Clinical examination and radiological features plus tumour excision and removal of some or all of the axillary lymph nodes give information about tumour stage. The TNM system of staging is commonly used – T [tumour size], N [involvement of lymph nodes], and M [distant metastases]. Imaging of other areas of the body (lungs, liver, bone) is often included at baseline. In reality it is relatively uncommon for breast cancer to present with spread beyond axillary lymph nodes [21]. Once breast cancer has spread beyond the locoregional lymph nodes, it is extremely unlikely to be cured. Both clinical and pathological features of a breast cancer have implications for prognosis and treatment.

5 Breast Cancer Treatment

Surgery: approaches to breast cancer management initially centred around mastectomy; however, it is now clear that since early-stage breast cancer patients are equally well treated with local wide excision and breast radiotherapy, the extent of surgery for a small breast cancer may be a matter of personal choice [22, 23]. Surgical excision of axillary lymph nodes is important for prognosis and to aid decisions about adjuvant therapy but more recently again the approach has moved towards sampling of nodes likely to be involved rather than removing all possible lymph nodes from the axilla [24].

Hormonal manipulation: since the earliest reports of the ability of even advanced breast cancer to respond to the removal of circulating oestrogen in 1896, oophorectomy and ovarian ablation to prevent oestrogen production in premenopausal women and pharmacological approaches to block oestrogen receptors or inhibit oestrogen production have been important strategies in breast cancer treatment [25]. It is now clear that in general only oestrogen receptor positive breast cancers are likely to respond to these approaches.

Cytotoxic therapies: Radiotherapy to the breast after breast conserving surgery and to the chest wall after mastectomy reduces the risk of local recurrence of breast cancer. The radiation field may be extended to include the axilla in some cases. Radiotherapy is also frequently used to reduce pain from bone metastases and symptoms from brain metastases when breast cancer spreads to distant sites.

Breast cancers are often sensitive to a wide range of cytotoxic chemotherapy drugs of the anthracycline type (anti-tumour antibiotics that interfere with enzymes involved in DNA replication) and increasingly now taxanes (mitotic spindle poisons) are included in many first-line adjuvant chemotherapy regimens. For high-grade and particularly ER-negative breast cancers, adjuvant cytotoxic chemotherapy is clearly beneficial in reducing the risk of distant spread of the disease [26].

Novel targeted therapies: As the pathological and molecular complexities of breast cancer are unravelled, opportunities arise for the development of novel therapies that are specifically aimed at blocking or suppressing tumour promoting pathways or mechanisms. One example of a very successful new biological targeted therapy is Herceptin which is an antibody to the HER2 receptor and is highly effective at reducing the risk of recurrence and at treating metastatic breast cancer for breast tumours in which the *HER2* gene is amplified [27].

6 Breast Cancer Genetics

Breast cancer is one of the commonest cancers in women in the western world. It is likely that all women who develop breast cancer have some genetic susceptibility.

Although only about 12% have one affected close relative, risk for breast cancer increases with increasing numbers of affected relatives [28]. This reflects the increasing likelihood of a high-penetrance dominant susceptibility gene segregating in a family with multiple affected close relatives. The majority of familial cases, however, are likely to be due to a combination of numerous common genetic variants that slightly increase the individual risk of breast cancer when compared to the population average (<1.5 fold increase per allele) [29]. These low-penetrance risk allele effects are likely to be multiplicative [30]. Rare mutations in other genes have also been implicated in relatively low-penetrance (two- to threefold increase) breast cancer susceptibility [31]. Only a rather small percentage of all cases (almost certainly less than 5%) are likely to be carriers of a high-risk susceptibility gene such as *BRCA1*, *BRCA2*, or *TP53* [3].

The average age of diagnosis of breast cancer in a white Caucasian population is around 60–65 years. Less than 20% of breast cancers are diagnosed under 50 years of age and only 5–10% under 40 years. The proportion of young onset breast cancers that are due to a highly penetrant single dominantly inherited breast cancer predisposition gene is higher than in later onset breast cancer cases [32, 33]. There is evidence of variation in the prevalence of pathological subtypes and the average age of onset of breast cancer in different age groups, in different geographical areas, and in different ethnic groups [16, 34]. These observations imply that genetic factors are important in breast cancer aetiology but that it is important to recognise that breast cancer is not a single disease entity, risk factors (including genetic risk factors) may vary for each different breast cancer subtype.

7 Gene Discovery

There are a variety of approaches that have been taken to identifying breast cancer predisposition genes, the chosen approach depends on the underlying genetic model and different methods allow the discovery of different types of genetic predisposition.

7.1 Linkage Analysis

Early breast cancer segregation analyses found that an autosomal dominant, rare, highly penetrant gene (or genes) was the most likely model that fit the available population data [1, 35]. Initial attempts to find breast cancer predisposition genes focused on familial multiple cases with early onset. The *TP53* gene was the first identified through the very striking clinical phenotype described by Li and Fraumeni [36–38], the *BRCA1* gene was mapped in the same year to chromosome 17 and *BRCA2* followed a few years later [39–42]. No further such high-penetrance genes have been identified to date [43]. There may be unique families with a dominantly transmitted mutation but traditional linkage studies using groups of families would not be able to detect such a gene. However, the majority of familial breast cancer clusters are now thought to be due to co-inheritance of multiple lower penetrance genetic variants. Genome-wide linkage analysis may be successful in detecting further loci of interest in familial cases [44].

7.2 Candidate Gene Resequencing

Examination of genotypes in familial cancer cases compared to population controls has become easier with the development of faster and more cost-effective molecular techniques. Taking a candidate gene approach, rare pathogenic mutations in several genes have been found at significantly higher frequencies in familial cases compared with controls. These are estimated to confer a modest increase in relative risk of developing breast cancer of the order of two to three times the population risk. The DNA repair genes have been particularly rewarding candidates for this type of investigation [45–47].

7.3 Genetic Association Studies

Following the success of linkage studies to identify rare mutations with a high penetrance in genes such as *TP53* and *BRCA1/2*, association studies have been used to identify common mutations with low risk. This statistical approach compares the frequency of single nucleotide polymorphisms (SNPs) in unrelated disease cases and healthy controls. SNPs with frequencies which differ significantly between cases and controls mark the vicinity of disease causing alterations, even if they themselves are not responsible. Genome-wide association (GWA) studies scan the entire genome for SNPs affecting a certain disease without a prior hypothesis of likely candidate genes or knowledge of disease pathogenesis. As a result of this unbiased approach, many novel pathways and genes have been identified that would not be candidates otherwise and may provide vital new insights and targets for therapeutic intervention.

To date, nine genes with relative risks of 1.1–1.9 have been identified by GWAs [30–54] which account for approximately 4% of familial risk when their effects are combined (Table 2.1). Further GWAs are currently underway and a second phase of the Wellcome Trust Case Control Consortium will provide genotypic data from 6,000 controls. However, even accounting for all known loci, including high-risk genes such as *BRCA1*, *BRCA2*, and *TP53* with relative risks of 5–10, at least 70% of the familial risk for breast cancer remains unexplained. Although the risk associated with some of the low penetrance loci may increase when causal rather than associated variants are determined, further loci undoubtedly remain to be detected. As genetic linkage studies have failed to identify further major breast cancer genes [43], much of the remaining genetic susceptibility is likely to be due to low-penetrance genes and perhaps rare genetic variants which are more suited to discovery by GWAs and sequencing than by linkage studies [55].

Table 2.1 Loci associated with breast cancer

Study	Cases	Controls	SNPs	Phenotype	Population	Associations	Odds ratio	P value
Easton et al. [30]	408	400	266, 722	Invasive, onset <60, positive family history, BRCA1/2 –ve	UK	FGFR2	1.26	4×10^{-16}
						TNRC9	1.11	10^{-7}
						MAP3K1	1.13	4×10^{-6}
						LSP1	1.07	8×10^{-6}
						H19	0.96	7×10^{-6}
						8q24.21	1.08	2×10^{-7}
Hunter et al. [48]	1, 183	1, 185	528, 173	Invasive, post-menopausal, sporadic	USA, self-reported Caucasian	FGFR2	1.23	1.2×10^{-5}
WTCCC [65]	1, 004	1, 464	15, 436	Invasive, positive family history, BRCA1/2 –ve	UK, self-reported Caucasian	MUC1[a]	1.25	1.3×10^{-4}
Stacey et al. [66]	1, 600	11, 563	311, 524	Invasive, median onset 56.3 years, 4.9% BRCA2	Iceland	TNRC9	1.23	4.7×10^{-6}
						2q35	1.19	9.2×10^{-6}
Kibriya et al. [67]	30	30	203, 477	Invasive, BRCA1/2 –ve	USA, Canada, Germany, Caucasian, Hispanic, African American	GLG1[a,b]	–	4.04×10^{-7}
						UGT1[a,b]	–	4.89×10^{-7}

Table 2.1 (continued)

Study	Cases	Controls	SNPs	Phenotype	Population	Associations	Odds ratio	P value
Gold et al. [50]	249	299	435, 632	Breast cancer, median onset 55, positive family history, BRCA1/2 –ve	USA, Canada, Israel, genetically isolated Ashkenazi Jews	FGFR2 6q22.33	1.26 1.41	1.5×10^{-5} 2.9×10^{-8}
Zheng et al. [54]	1, 505	1, 522	607, 728	Breast cancer	Chinese	6q25.1 ESR1	1.56	1.4×10^{-5}
Cox et al. [68]	16, 423 12, 946	17, 109 15, 109	9	Invasive, sporadic and positive family history	18 European and two Asian populations	CASP8 TGFB1	0.88 1.08	5.7×10^{-7} 1.5×10^{-4}

[a]Not replicated
[b]Results from haplotype test

7.3.1 Breast Cancer Heterogeneity

Breast cancer is a heterogeneous disease that can be subdivided on the basis of conventional histology and immunohistochemical markers [56, 57] and gene expression profiles [13, 15]. The gene expression subsets are largely determined by levels of hormone receptor-related genes such as *ER*, *PR*, and *HER2* and, therefore, overlap largely with the histological subsets. For example, most basal-like subtypes of breast cancer are triple-negative breast cancer (ER–ve, PR–ve, HER2–ve). Luminal subtypes are typically ER positive. These subtypes of breast cancer are increasingly recognised as separate diseases with different outcomes [58]. Increasingly different treatment approaches are being considered for specific subtypes of breast cancer [59]. Characteristic morphological features have been highlighted in *BRCA1*, *BRCA2*, and other familial breast cancer groups [60–62]. Unsurprisingly perhaps, breast cancers arising in high-risk gene carriers can also be demonstrated to broadly share molecular characteristics using a variety of genomic techniques [63, 64].

7.3.2 Common Genetic Variants and Breast Cancer Phenotype

Recent studies have demonstrated that some of the associations between common genetic variants and the risk of developing breast cancer are probably specific to certain subgroups, broadly at the moment observed when ER-negative and ER-positive breast cancers are considered as separate groups [49, 66, 69]. This supports the concept that subtypes of breast cancer have different genetic components of risk. Many GWAs have failed to accounted for this heterogeneity which may have reduced their power and explain some of the failures to replicate previous findings [70]. Confining GWAs to subsets of breast cancer that show a strong component of genetic risk (by selecting cases with positive family histories) or a specific subgroup of breast tumour type will reduce genetic heterogeneity and increase power to detect subtype specific effects and novel genes.

7.3.3 Common Genetic Variants and Prognosis

Recent studies have suggested that the prognosis of breast cancer is also influenced by genetic factors. The process of tumour development and progression varies considerably between patients. The known tumour features that are used to predict prognosis are noted at the time of presentation – tumour size, grade, ER status, HER2 status, locoregional lymph node involvement, etc. A variety of prognostic algorithms are used clinically to predict risk of relapse, new molecular profiles are being tested [10, 71, 72]. None predict with certainty for an individual and it is realistic to expect that individual genetic background will affect response to tumour growth and metastasis as well as to risk. Recent data from a population-based study indicated that daughters and sisters of a proband with poor prognosis had a 60% higher 5-year breast cancer mortality compared to those of a proband with good prognosis (hazard ratio 1.6, P for trend 0.002), suggesting an inherited component to prognosis [73].

In a pilot study to explore the role of common genetic variants in breast cancer prognosis, 30 candidate genes were selected for investigation. Tagging SNPs across the 30 candidate genes were typed in 1,001 individuals from the Prospective study of Outcomes in Sporadic versus Hereditary breast cancer (POSH) cohort, three genes were identified that influence distant disease-free survival (DDFS) times and these effects are independent of tumour-specific factors [74] (Fig. 2.3). To date, however, there have been no GWAs to identify genes that influence outcome after diagnosis of breast cancer.

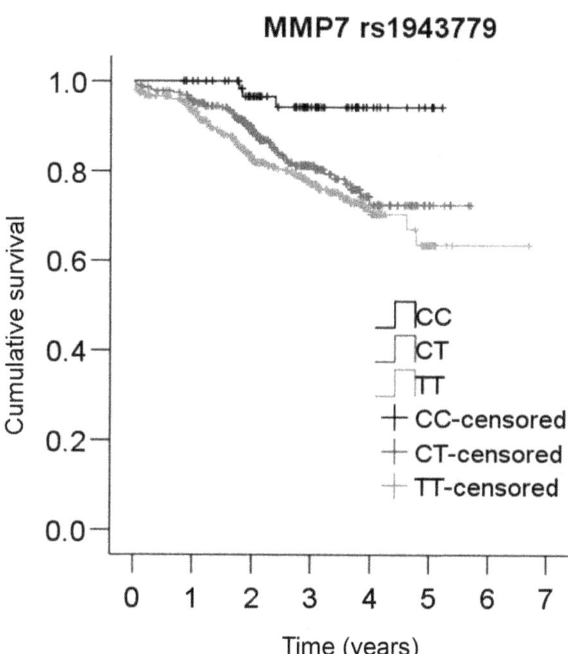

Fig. 2.3 Kaplan Meir survival analysis showing that the genotype of SNP rs1943779 in the MMP7 gene is sigificantly associated with the chance of relapsing after a breast cancer diagnosis

7.3.4 Host Response to Treatment

Pharmacogenetics is the study of genetic variants that influence the response to drugs, for example by affecting the rate and efficiency of drug metabolism. Clearly then genetic variation may well influence prognosis since in many cases the prognosis of the individual is being influenced by the treatment administered. In diseases other than breast cancer, genetic factors have been demonstrated to affect the efficacy of treatments by altering their absorption and receptor-ligand interactions [75]. In breast cancer, a recent study has shown that genetic variants of CYP2D6 and CYP2C19 may influence prognosis by altering the metabolism and subsequent efficacy of tamoxifen in ER-positive breast cancer; however, the evidence is conflicting

[76, 77]. Mutations of NQO1 have also been shown to influence prognosis in breast cancer by impairing the response of patients to epirubicin but this observation has not yet been confirmed by others [78].

7.3.5 Breast Cancer Growth and Metastases in the Host Environment

Breast cancers arise due to the accumulation of multiple genetic and epigenetic perturbations that enhance the growth and division capability of the cell of origin. More rapid proliferation in the absence of any of the important regulatory mechanisms increases the likelihood of cellular DNA acquiring new somatic and epigenetic mutations during replication. Loss of normal mechanisms for DNA repair and for apoptosis (programmed cell death) leads to disordered growth and eventually the accumulation of more mutations enhancing the ability of the tumour to invade and metastasise which are the hallmarks of a malignant tumour. Several mechanisms may be important for preventing malignancy and many of these are under genetic control. The immune system, DNA repair genes, and host stromal elements (e.g. matrix metalloproteinases) are all good biological candidates for a potential role in individually variable responses to tumourigenesis and the development and growth of metastases. Breast cancers typically spread to bone, brain, lung, and liver, but the site of metastasis is unpredictable even when similar tumours are compared. Germline polymorphisms have been shown to contribute to these variations in the site of metastasis [79]. In human breast cancer, inherited polymorphisms in Brd4 and Sipa1 (with which Brd4 interacts) have been shown to alter protein expression and are predictive of metastasis and increased expression of TNRC9 is associated with metastasis to bone [80–82].

7.3.6 Challenges in Genome-Wide Association Studies

Despite the success of GWAs many limitations and challenges remain. Many of the susceptibility alleles identified are so common that a high proportion of the general population are carriers with small risk. It is, therefore, unlikely that these SNPs will be appropriate for predictive testing until the estimated risk associated with them is increased by identifying causal alleles or combinations of associated variants [83, 84]. Once a variant has been reproducibly associated with disease the next step is to perform functional studies that identify causal mutation(s), which may differ from the associated variant and which may lead to potential new avenues for therapeutic intervention. Functional analyses aim to demonstrate that causal mutations alter the expression or function of a gene resulting in biologically plausible consequences. For example, a comprehensive study of CTLA4 variants in autoimmune disease demonstrated that the causal allele is located in the regulatory 3′ untranslated region of the gene rather than the leader peptide which contained the associated variant [85].

In order for future GWAs to detect further susceptibility loci, it is anticipated that larger numbers of cases and controls will be required. This may be achieved as genotyping costs fall and as more large consortia come together to combine data across multiple studies. Previous GWAs of breast cancer have relied on approximately 15,000–530,000 SNPs to capture information from an estimated 7–15 million SNPs in the genome through linkage disequilibrium (LD). In some regions, however, the coverage is incomplete resulting in a loss of power to detect associated variants in these areas. Following completion of phase II of the HapMap project, which characterised over 3.1 million SNPs [86], and the introduction of high-density chips that contain over 2 million SNPs and copy number variations, new GWAs will provide more comprehensive scans of the genome that will lead to the identification of novel susceptibility genes.

In general, association studies are required to note the ethnicity of cases and controls and minimise bias due to the selection/matching of particular individuals from a wider population since population stratification can lead to false positives. This is especially true for breast cancer which appears to be more severe in women with African ancestry [87]. Prior to the analysis of GWA data, it is therefore prudent to test the homogeneity of the sample and exclude any outliers. The PLINK program [88] uses a multidimensional scaling analysis of genome-wide average identities by state (IBS) and with additional data from Caucasian, African, and Asian populations from the HapMap project [86] was used, for example, to assess ethnic homogeneity in 1,001 British breast cancer cases prior to association testing [74]. Plotting the first two components from the multidimensional scaling analysis, which represent geographic and genetic variation, clearly identified three distinct clusters that correspond to African, Asian, and Western European ancestries (Fig. 2.4). This information was used to ensure that variation in SNP profiles resulting from

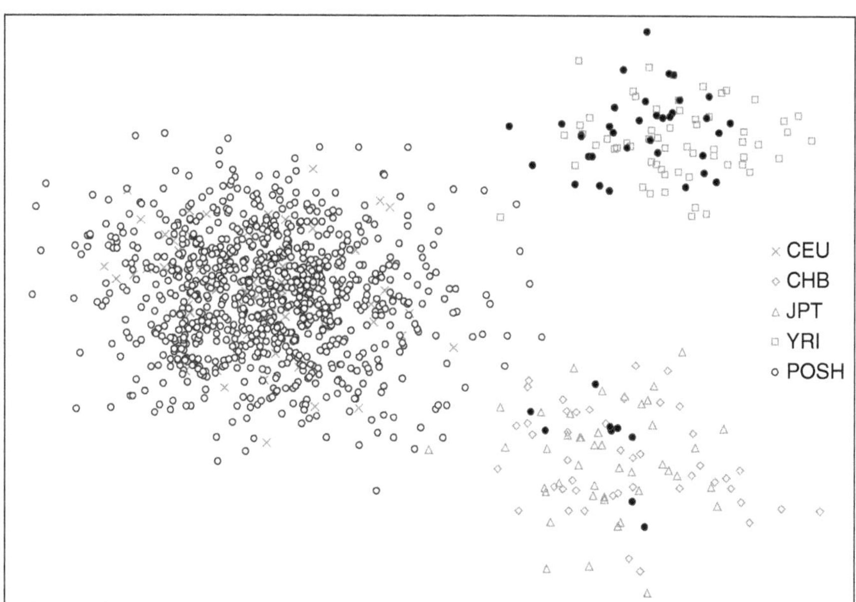

Fig. 2.4 Identifying evidence of population stratification

different ethnic backgrounds were not confounding the analysis of SNPs associated with disease characteristics [74].

GWAs were developed with the hypothesis that common diseases, such as breast cancer, are caused by common, low-penetrance variants. However, if rarer variants with higher penetrance are responsible, future GWAs will need to genotype more people and SNPs to detect this type of variant and genome-wide linkage analysis may be an alternative approach [44]. By sequencing the genomes of 1,000 people, the 1,000 genomes project aims to produce a genome-wide map of variations found in 1% of the population, 10 times rarer than those provided by the HapMap project. This project will also characterise structural variations of the genome such as rearrangements, deletions, or duplications of the genome which may play a role in susceptibility to diseases. This information will facilitate the detection of causal variants by identifying almost all variants in a region associated with disease and helping to select variants for functional studies.

8 Summary

The study of genetic influences in breast cancer is complex. Careful case selection is important with account being taken of ethnic homogeneity, disease phenotype, and environmental risk factor exposure. The translation of current knowledge about common polymorphisms and breast cancer susceptibility has potential for early detection and risk stratification in future. Targeted breast cancer management strategies may require not only tumour molecular profiling but also knowledge of an individual's genetic susceptibility to develop metastatic disease. There is still a great deal more that needs to be discovered and understood before this type of genetic knowledge will find a valid place in clinical care of individuals and families with breast cancer.

References

1. Claus EB, Risch N, Thompson WD (1991) Genetic analysis of breast cancer in the cancer and steroid hormone study. Am J Hum Genet 48(2):232–242
2. Hartman M, Hall P, Edgren G et al (2008) Breast cancer onset in twins and women with bilateral disease. J Clin Oncol 26(25):4086–4091
3. Stratton MR, Rahman N (2008) The emerging landscape of breast cancer susceptibility. Nat Genet 40(1):17–22
4. Antoniou AC, Hardy R, Walker L et al (2008) Predicting the likelihood of carrying a BRCA1 or BRCA2 mutation: validation of BOADICEA, BRCAPRO, IBIS, Myriad and the Manchester scoring system using data from UK genetics clinics. J Med Genet 45(7):425–431
5. Ford D, Easton DF, Stratton M et al (1998) Genetic heterogeneity and penetrance analysis of the BRCA1 and BRCA2 genes in breast cancer families. The Breast Cancer Linkage Consortium. Am J Hum Genet 62(3):676–689
6. Antoniou AC, Spurdle AB, Sinilnikova OM et al (2008) Common breast cancer-predisposition alleles are associated with breast cancer risk in BRCA1 and BRCA2 mutation carriers. Am J Hum Genet 82(4):937–948

7. Wiseman RA (2004) Breast cancer: critical data analysis concludes that estrogens are not the cause, however lifestyle changes can alter risk rapidly. J Clin Epidemiol 57(8):766–772
8. Ziegler RG, Hoover RN, Pike MC et al (1993) Migration patterns and breast cancer risk in Asian-American women. J Natl Cancer Inst 85(22):1819–1827
9. Pakkiri P, Lakhani SR, Smart CE (2009) Current and future approach to the pathologist's assessment for targeted therapy in breast cancer. Pathology 41(1):89–99
10. Galea MH, Blamey RW, Elston CE, Ellis IO (1992) The Nottingham prognostic index in primary breast cancer. Breast Cancer Res Treat 22:207–219
11. Schmidt M, Victor A, Bratzel D et al (2008) Long-term outcome prediction by clinicopathological risk classification algorithms in node-negative breast cancer – comparison between Adjuvant! St Gallen, and a novel risk algorithm used in the prospective randomized Node-Negative-Breast Cancer-3 (NNBC-3) trial. Ann Oncol 20(2):258–264
12. Piccart-Gebhart MJ, Procter M, Leyland-Jones B et al (2005) Trastuzumab after adjuvant chemotherapy in HER2-positive breast cancer. N Engl J Med 353(16):1659–1672
13. Sorlie T, Perou CM, Tibshirani R et al (2001) Gene expression patterns of breast carcinomas distinguish tumor subclasses with clinical implications. Proc Natl Acad Sci USA 98:10869–10874
14. Wessels LF, van Welsem T, Hart AA, van't Veer LJ, Reinders MJ, Nederlof PM (2002) Molecular classification of breast carcinomas by comparative genomic hybridization: a specific somatic genetic profile for BRCA1 tumors. Cancer Res 62(23):7110–7117
15. Perou CM, Sorlie T, Eisen MB et al (2000) Molecular portraits of human breast tumours. Nature 406:747–752
16. Anderson WF, Rosenberg PS, Menashe I, Mitani A, Pfeiffer RM (2008) Age-related crossover in breast cancer incidence rates between black and white ethnic groups. J Natl Cancer Inst 100(24):1804–1814
17. Bowen RL, Duffy SW, Ryan DA, Hart IR, Jones JL (2008) Early onset of breast cancer in a group of British black women. Br J Cancer 98(2):277–281
18. Anderson WF, Chu KC, Chang S, Sherman ME (2004) Comparison of age-specific incidence rate patterns for different histopathologic types of breast carcinoma. Cancer Epidemiol Biomarkers Prev 13(7):1128–1135
19. Walker RA, Lees E, Webb MB, Dearing SJ (1996) Breast carcinomas occurring in young women (<35 years) are different. Br J Cancer 74(11):1796–1800
20. Lakhani SR, Reis-Filho JS, Fulford L et al (2005) Prediction of BRCA1 status in patients with breast cancer using estrogen receptor and basal phenotype. Clin Cancer Res 11(14): 5175–5180
21. Sobin LH (2003) TNM, sixth edition: new developments in general concepts and rules. Semin Surg Oncol 21:19–22
22. Veronesi U, Salvadori B, Luini A et al (1995) Breast-conservation is a safe method in patients with small cancer of the breast – long-term results of 3 randomized trials on 1,973 patients. Eur J Cancer 31A(10):1574–1579
23. Throckmorton AD, Esserman LJ (2009) When informed, all women do not prefer breast conservation. J Clin Oncol 27(4):484–486
24. Gui GP, Joubert DJ, Reichert R et al (2005) Continued axillary sampling is unnecessary and provides no further information to sentinel node biopsy in staging breast cancer. Eur J Surg Oncol 31(7):707–714
25. Piccart-Gebhart MJ (2004) New stars in the sky of treatment for early breast cancer. N Engl J Med 350(11):1140–1142
26. Clarke M (2006) Meta-analyses of adjuvant therapies for women with early breast cancer: the Early Breast Cancer Trialists' Collaborative Group overview. Ann Oncol 17(Supplement 10):x59–x62
27. Untch M, Gelber RD, Jackisch C et al (2008) Estimating the magnitude of trastuzumab effects within patient subgroups in the HERA trial. Ann Oncol 19(6):1090–1096
28. Collaborative Group on Hormonal Factors in Breast Cancer (2001) Familial breast cancer: collaborative reanalysis of individual data from 52 epidemiological studies including

58,209 women with breast cancer and 101,986 women without the disease. Lancet 358(9291):1389–1399

29. Pharoah PD, Antoniou A, Bobrow M, Zimmern RL, Easton DF, Ponder BA (2002) Polygenic susceptibility to breast cancer and implications for prevention. Nat Genet 31(1):33–36

30. Easton DF, Pooley KA, Dunning AM et al (2007) Genome-wide association study identifies novel breast cancer susceptibility loci. Nature 447(7148):1087–1093

31. Walsh T, King MC (2007) Ten genes for inherited breast cancer. Cancer Cell 11(2):103–105

32. Lalloo F, Varley J, Moran A et al (2006) BRCA1, BRCA2 and TP53 mutations in very early-onset breast cancer with associated risks to relatives. Eur J Cancer 42(8):1143–1150

33. Bonadona V, Sinilnikova OM, Chopin S et al (2005) Contribution of BRCA1 and BRCA2 germ-line mutations to the incidence of breast cancer in young women: results from a prospective population-based study in France. Genes Chromosomes Cancer 43(4):404–413

34. Anderson WF, Chen BE, Brinton LA, Devesa SS (2007) Qualitative age interactions (or effect modification) suggest different cancer pathways for early-onset and late-onset breast cancers. Cancer Causes Control 18(10):1187–1198

35. Eccles D, Marlow A, Royle G, Collins A, Morton NE (1994) Genetic epidemiology of early onset breast cancer. J Med Genet 31(12):944–949

36. Li FP, Fraumeni JFJ (1969) Soft-tissue sarcomas, breast cancer, and other neoplasms. A familial syndrome? Ann Intern Med 71(4):747–752

37. Li FP, Fraumeni JF Jr, Mulvihill JJ et al (1988) A cancer family syndrome in twenty-four kindreds. Cancer Res 48(18):5358–5362

38. Malkin D, Li FP, Strong LC et al (1990) Germ line p53 mutations in a familial syndrome of breast cancer, sarcomas, and other neoplasms. Science 250(4985):1233–1238

39. Hall JM, Lee MK, Newman B et al (1990) Linkage of early-onset familial breast cancer to chromosome 17q21. Science 250(4988):1684–1689

40. Miki Y, Swensen J, Shattuck-Eidens D et al (1994) A strong candidate for the breast and ovarian cancer susceptibility gene BRCA1. Science 266(5182):66–71

41. Wooster R, Neuhausen SL, Mangion J et al (1994) Localization of a breast cancer suscepti-bility gene, BRCA2, to chromosome 13q12-13. Science 265(5181):2088–2090

42. Wooster R, Bignell G, Lancaster J et al (1995) Identification of the breast cancer susceptibility gene BRCA2. Nature 378(6559):789–792

43. Smith P, McGuffog L, Easton DF et al (2006) A genome wide linkage search for breast cancer susceptibility genes. Genes Chromosomes Cancer 45(7):646–655

44. Rosa-Rosa JM, Pita G, Urioste M et al (2009) Genome-wide linkage scan reveals three putative breast-cancer-susceptibility loci. Am J Hum Genet 84(2):115–122

45. Renwick A, Thompson D, Seal S et al (2006) ATM mutations that cause ataxia-telangiectasia are breast cancer susceptibility alleles. Nat Genet 38(8):873–875

46. Rahman N, Seal S, Thompson D et al (2007) PALB2, which encodes a BRCA2-interacting protein, is a breast cancer susceptibility gene. Nat Genet 39(2):165–167

47. Seal S, Thompson D, Renwick A et al (2006) Truncating mutations in the Fanconi ane-mia J gene BRIP1 are low-penetrance breast cancer susceptibility alleles. Nat Genet 38(11): 1239–1241

48. Hunter DJ, Kraft P, Jacobs KB et al (2007) A genome-wide association study identifies alleles in FGFR2 associated with risk of sporadic postmenopausal breast cancer. Nat Genet 39(7):870–874

49. Stacey SN, Manolescu A, Sulem P et al (2008) Common variants on chromosome 5p12 confer susceptibility to estrogen receptor-positive breast cancer. Nat Genet 40(6):703–706

50. Gold B, Kirchhoff T, Stefanov S et al (2008) Genome-wide association study provides evi-dence for a breast cancer risk locus at 6q22-33. Proc Natl Acad Sci USA 105(11):4340–4345

51. Argos M, Kibriya MG, Jasmine F et al (2008) Genomewide scan for loss of heterozygosity and chromosomal amplification in breast carcinoma using single-nucleotide polymorphism arrays. Cancer Genet Cytogenet 182(2):69–74

52. Newport M, Sirugo G, Lyons E et al (2007) Association scan of 14,500 nonsynonymous SNPs in four diseases identifies autoimmunity variants. Nat Genet 39(11):1329–1337

53. Kibriya MG, Jasmine F, Argos M et al (2009) A pilot genome-wide association study of early-onset breast cancer. Breast Cancer Res Treat 114(3):463–477
54. Zheng W, Long JR, Gao YT et al (2009) Genome-wide association study identifies a new breast cancer susceptibility locus at 6q25.1. Nat Genet 41(3):324–328
55. Risch N, Merikangas K (1996) The future of genetic studies of complex human diseases. Science 273(5281):1516–1517
56. Abd El-Rehim DM, Pinder SE, Paish CE et al (2004) Expression of luminal and basal cytokeratins in human breast carcinoma. J Pathol 203(2):661–671
57. Makretsov NA, Huntsman DG, Nielsen TO et al (2004) Hierarchical clustering analysis of tissue microarray immunostaining data identifies prognostically significant groups of breast carcinoma. Clin Cancer Res 10(18 Pt 1):6143–6151
58. Sorlie T, Tibshirani R, Parker J et al (2003) Repeated observation of breast tumor subtypes in independent gene expression data sets. Proc Natl Acad Sci USA 100:8418–8423
59. Turner NC, Reis-Filho JS, Russell AM et al (2007) BRCA1 dysfunction in sporadic basal-like breast cancer. Oncogene 26(14):2126–2132
60. Lakhani SR (1999) The pathology of familial breast cancer: morphological aspects. Breast Cancer Res 1(1):31–35
61. Lakhani SR, Van D V, Jacquemier J et al (2002) The pathology of familial breast cancer: predictive value of immunohistochemical markers estrogen receptor, progesterone receptor, HER-2, and p53 in patients with mutations in BRCA1 and BRCA2. J Clin Oncol 20(9): 2310–2318
62. Palacios J, Honrado E, Osorio A et al (2005) Phenotypic characterization of BRCA1 and BRCA2 tumors based in a tissue microarray study with 37 immunohistochemical markers. Breast Cancer Res Treat 90(1):5–14
63. Hedenfalk IA, Ringner M, Trent JM, Borg A (2002) Gene expression in inherited breast cancer. Adv Cancer Res 84:1–34
64. Jonsson G, Naylor TL, Vallon-Christersson J et al (2005) Distinct genomic profiles in hereditary breast tumors identified by array-based comparative genomic hybridization. Cancer Res 65(17):7612–7621
65. The Wellcome Trust Case Control Consortium (2007) Genome-wide association study of 14,000 cases of seven common diseases and 3,000 shared controls. Nature 447:661–678
66. Stacey SN, Manolescu A, Sulem P et al (2007) Common variants on chromosomes 2q35 and 16q12 confer susceptibility to estrogen receptor-positive breast cancer. Nat Genet 39(7): 865–869
67. Kibriya MG, Jasmine F, Argos M et al (2009) A pilot genome-wide association study of early-onset breast cancer. Breast Cancer Res Treat 114(3):463–477
68. Cox A, Dunning AM, Garcia-Closas M, Balasubramanian S et al (2007) A common coding variant in CASP8 is associated with breast cancer risk. Nat Genet 39(3):352–358
69. Garcia-Closas M, Hall P, Nevanlinna H et al (2008) Heterogeneity of breast cancer associations with five susceptibility loci by clinical and pathological characteristics. PLoS Genet 4(4):e1000054
70. Amos CI (2007) Successful design and conduct of genome-wide association studies. Hum Mol Genet 16(R2):R220–R225
71. Ozanne EM, Braithwaite D, Sepucha K, Moore D, Esserman L, Belkora J (2009) Sensitivity to input variability of the adjuvant! Online breast cancer prognostic model. J Clin Oncol 27(2):214–219
72. Bueno-de-Mesquita JM, van Harten WH, Retel VP et al (2007) Use of 70-gene signature to predict prognosis of patients with node-negative breast cancer: a prospective community-based feasibility study (RASTER). Lancet Oncol 8(12):1079–1087
73. Hartman M, Lindstrom L, Dickman PW, Adami HO, Hall P, Czene K (2007) Is breast cancer prognosis inherited? Breast Cancer Res 9(3):R39
74. Tapper W, Hammond V, Gerty S et al (2008) The influence of genetic variation in thirty selected genes on the clinical characteristics of early onset breast cancer. Breast Cancer Res 10(6):R108

75. Liu ZL, He B, Fang F, Tang CY, Zou LP (2008) Genetic polymorphisms of MC2R gene associated with responsiveness to adrenocorticotropic hormone therapy in infantile spasms. Chinese Med J 121(17):1627–1632
76. Schroth W, Antoniadou L, Fritz P et al (2007) Breast cancer treatment outcome with adjuvant tamoxifen relative to patient CYP2D6 and CYP2C19 genotypes. J Clin Oncol 25(33): 5187–5193
77. Okishiro M, Taguchi T, Kim SJ, Shimazu K, Tamaki Y, Noguchi S (2009) Genetic polymorphisms of CYP2D6*10 and CYP2C19*2,*3 are not associated with prognosis, endometrial thickness, or bone mineral density in Japanese breast cancer patients treated with adjuvant tamoxifen. Cancer 115(5):952–961
78. Fagerholm R, Hofstetter B, Tommiska J et al (2008) NAD(P)H:quinone oxidoreductase 1 NQO1*2 genotype (P187S) is a strong prognostic and predictive factor in breast cancer. Nat Genet 40(7):844–853
79. Hsieh SM, Lintell NA, Hunter KW (2006) Germline polymorphisms are potential metastasis risk and prognosis markers in breast cancer. Breast Dis 26:157–162
80. Crawford NPS, Alsarraj J, Lukes L et al (2008) Bromodomain 4 activation predicts breast cancer survival. Proc Natl Acad Sci USA 105(17):6380–6385
81. Park YG, Zhao XH, Lesueur F et al (2005) Sipa1 is a candidate for underlying the metastasis efficiency modifier locus Mtes1. Nat Genet 37(10):1055–1062
82. Smid M, Wang Y, Klijn JG et al (2006) Genes associated with breast cancer metastatic to bone. J Clin Oncol 24(15):2261–2267
83. Gail MH (2008) Discriminatory accuracy from single-nucleotide polymorphisms in models to predict breast cancer risk. J Natl Cancer Inst 100(14):1037–1041
84. Pharoah PD, Antoniou AC, Easton DF, Ponder BA (2008) Polygenes, risk prediction, and targeted prevention of breast cancer. N Engl J Med 358(26):2796–2803
85. Ueda H, Howson JM, Esposito L et al (2003) Association of the T-cell regulatory gene CTLA4 with susceptibility to autoimmune disease. Nature 423(6939):506–511
86. Gibbs RA, Belmont JW, Hardenbol P et al (2003) The international HapMap project. Nature 426(6968):789–796
87. Bowen RL, Stebbing J, Jones LJ (2006) A review of the ethnic differences in breast cancer. Pharmacogenomics 7(6):935–942
88. Purcell S, Neale B, Todd-Brown K et al (2007) PLINK: a tool set for whole-genome association and population-based linkage analyses. Am J Hum Genet 81(3):559–575

Chapter 3
Hereditary Diffuse Gastric Cancer

Kasmintan Schrader and David Huntsman

Abstract Gastric cancer is one of the world's leading causes of cancer mortality. A small percentage of cases can be attributed to heritable mutations in highly penetrant cancer susceptibility genes. In this chapter we will focus on the genetic cause of hereditary diffuse gastric cancer (HDGC). Until 10 years ago, individuals from these families lived with the uncertainty of developing lethal gastric cancer. Today, HDGC families can be identified, tested for causative mutations in *CDH1*, and for those families where a pathogenic mutation can be identified, prophylactic total gastrectomy can be implemented in asymptomatic mutation carriers who elect to virtually eliminate their risk of developing this lethal disease.

Hereditary diffuse gastric cancer (HDGC) is an autosomal dominant familial cancer syndrome characterized by multiple cases of early-onset diffuse gastric cancer. *CDH1* is the only gene that has been associated with HDGC [1] where the risk of developing clinically significant diffuse gastric cancer (DGC) is 63–83% and 40–67% for male and female mutation carriers, respectively [2, 3].

CDH1 encodes E-cadherin, which is a cell-surface, transmembrane, glycoprotein that is critical for the adhesion of epithelial cells to each other. Loss of expression of E-cadherin has been associated with invasiveness of cancer cells. The majority of sporadic and hereditary DGC do not express E-cadherin, implying that mutation, loss, or methylation occurs to the normal *CDH1* alleles.

It might be expected that carriers of germline mutations in *CDH1* would be susceptible to further, different types of tumors. Indeed, in these families there is an additional 39–52% lifetime risk of developing breast cancer in females [2, 3]. The lobular breast cancer (LBC) subtype is associated with HDGC. This is consistent with the characteristic loss of E-cadherin expression in sporadic LBC [4–6].

K. Schrader (✉)

Department of Pathology and Laboratory Medicine and Department of Medical Genetics, University of British Columbia, British Columbia Cancer Agency, Vancouver, BC, Canada V5Z 4E6

e-mail: ischrader@bccancer.bc.ca

B. Pasche (ed.), *Cancer Genetics*, Cancer Treatment and Research 155,
DOI 10.1007/978-1-4419-6033-7_3, © Springer Science+Business Media, LLC 2010

The anatomical and histological appearance of DGC, which infiltrates the gastric wall beneath an apparently normal mucosa, is consistent with the loss of expression of E-cadherin. This normal appearance of the mucosa accounts for the difficulty in detecting disease in asymptomatic patients using endoscopy. Furthermore, DGC frequently metastasizes and once clinically symptomatic has a very poor survival rate. The identification of germline *CDH1* mutations as a cause in a large proportion of HDGC families has provided a significant clinical benefit. Thus, genetic testing of HDGC families for *CDH1* mutations enables unaffected mutation carriers to be selected for focused screening and consideration for the recommended prophylactic surgery, which is total gastrectomy. Prophylactic total gastrectomy (PTG) carries its own risks of morbidity and mortality; however, this is balanced by the lethality and insidious nature of DGC. It is currently the only unequivocal way to reduce the risk of DGC in carriers of germline *CDH1* mutations.

Prophylactic total gastrectomy has provided new insight and further challenges to the understanding of the natural history of DGC disease progression. Multiple microscopic foci of invasive DGC have been identified in the gastrectomy specimens of 69 out of 70 asymptomatic mutation carriers [5, 7–19]. Therefore, among these carriers, there has been almost complete penetrance of asymptomatic DGC. As penetrance data demonstrate that ~30% of *CDH1* carriers are not diagnosed with DGC over their lifetime, this implies that not all microscopic foci of intramucosal cancers become clinically significant. Nevertheless, as the biological mechanisms that underlie this ominous progression are not fully understood, PTG is recommended for germline *CDH1* mutation carriers as it remains the only unambiguous strategy to reduce the risk of DGC. In this review the pathology, epidemiology, and molecular genetics of GC and our current understanding of HDGC will be summarized.

1 Gastric Cancer Pathology, Epidemiology, and Molecular Genetics

1.1 Pathological Classification of Gastric Cancer

Adenocarcinomas comprise the vast majority of primary gastric cancer (GC). Multiple histological classification systems for adenocarcinomas have been developed to better predict their prognosis; however, for the purpose of defining genetic risk, the most useful system is the classification of Lauren [20]. This system classifies the majority of adenocarcinomas into two main types: the intestinal type and the diffuse type, with the remainder forming an indeterminate category [20]. Tumors with components of both types are classified as mixed [20].

The more common, intestinal type of gastric cancer (IGC) [21] is composed of glandular structures resembling intestinal epithelium. IGC arises from its precursor lesion, intestinal metaplasia [22], to form an exophytic tumor, which ulcerates the stomach lining. Due to its localized presentation and distinctive appearance, IGC tends to be amenable to detection by endoscopic surveillance.

In contrast, DGC shows scattered, disorganized growth without distinctive architecture. Malignant cells infiltrate the wall of the stomach, gradually thickening it so that it takes on a *leather bottle* appearance, otherwise known as *linitus plastica*. The neoplastic cells have a distinctive signet ring appearance caused by an accumulation of intracellular mucin that pushes the nucleus to one side. This is demonstrated in Fig. 3.1 where Fig. 3.1a shows the signet ring appearance with a regular hematoxylin and eosin (H&E) stain. These cells can be confused with small blood vessels that have been sectioned transversely; however, staining with PAS-D easily highlights the mucin-containing signet ring cells (Fig. 3.1c). Unlike IGC, DGC has no defined premalignant lesion, although, as noted, analysis of almost all reported PTG specimens has demonstrated multiple microscopic foci of invasive DGC [5, 7–19]. The DGC lesions associated with HDGC are usually very small and intramucosal, in situ or with pagetoid spread of signet ring cells [23]. These very small (<3mm) superficial clusters of invasive cancer are predominantly composed of signet ring cells and appear to follow a more indolent course [24]. What causes these small invasive cancers to become clinically significant is not fully understood; however, the phenotype of the DGC cells which spread beyond the mucosa is that of poor differentiation and activation of a known epithelial–mesenchymal transition inducer, Src kinase [24].

The Lauren classification of DGC is analogous to the Carneiro classification system's isolated cell type, as it is to the World Health Organization's classification of signet ring cell type [25]. Pathology reports indicating undifferentiated, mucinous adenocarcinoma or poorly differentiated adenocarcinomas also raise the index of suspicion for DGC. DGC typically exhibits decreased or absent immunohistochemical staining for E-cadherin, consistent with its disorganized architecture (Fig. 3.1b). Recognition of families with an autosomal dominant predisposition toward DGC led to the discovery of causative germline mutations in *CDH1* [1]. To date, *CDH1*

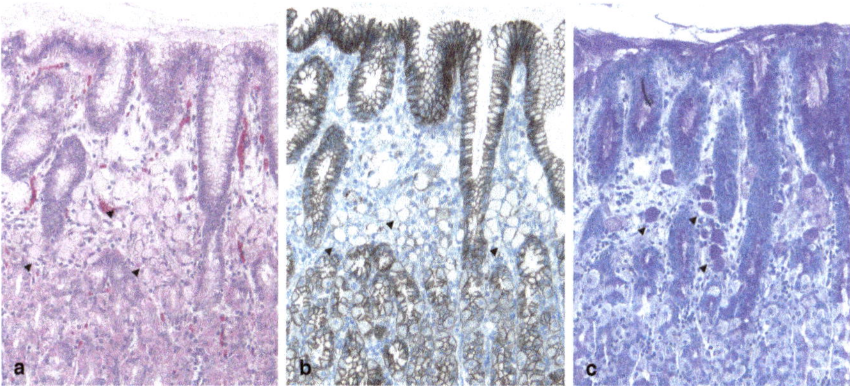

Fig. 3.1 These pictures show a small invasive focus of a diffuse gastric cancer from a prophylactic gastrectomy specimen: (**a**) H&E stain; (**b**) E-cadherin stain showing down-regulated expression in the invasive signet ring cells in comparison to the normal E-cadherin-positive epithelium; (**c**) PAS-D stain for mucin showing the presence of intracellular mucin in the cytoplasm of signet ring cells. Photographs taken by Dr Martin Köbel

remains the only gene associated with HDGC; likewise, germline aberrations in *CDH1* are exclusive to the syndrome, emphasizing the importance of the pathologic classification of these tumors.

1.2 Epidemiology of the Two Types of Gastric Cancer

The differences between the two types of GC extend beyond their morphologic appearances to their risk factors and patient demographics. As compared with DGC, the incidence of IGC increases more with age and affects males more than females. Worldwide there is marked variation in the incidence of GC and the proportion of the two subtypes. The highest rates of GC are found in Japan, China, Eastern Europe, and South America and the lowest in North America, Northern Europe, Southeastern Asian, and Northern and Western Africa. IGC comprises the majority of GC diagnoses in higher incidence countries, while DGC forms a higher proportion of GC cases in lower as compared to higher incidence countries.

Environmental factors contributing more to the development of IGC are thought to be responsible for these disparities. Chronic gastric mucosal infection with *Helicobacter pylori* leading to a chronic atrophic gastritis [27, 28] is the most well-recognized environmental risk factor for GC, with a relative risk of 5.9 for non-cardia GC [29]. Compared to the vast global rates of *H. pylori* infection, only a relatively small proportion of infected individuals go on to develop GC. This reflects the influence of genetic factors in the bacteria and the host. For example, strains of *H. pylori* containing the virulence factor cytotoxin-associated gene A (cagA) are carcinogenic [30]. CagA is a secreted bacterial oncoprotein introduced into gastric epithelial cells by bacterial secretion machinery [31]. When phosphorylated by Src or Abl kinase, it deregulates the tyrosine phosphatase Src homology-related protein (SHP-2), which acts upstream of the oncogenic Ras MAP kinase pathway [32]. Genetic variations in the host, such as particular polymorphisms in genes for the inflammatory mediators IL-1β, IL-1 receptor antagonist, TNF-α, IL-10, and IFNγR1 [33–35], dictate the type of immune and inflammatory response triggered by *H. pylori* infection. These bacterial and host genetic factors contribute to the progression of gastritis to chronic atrophic gastritis, to intestinal metaplasia, and finally GC. Additionally other environmental factors such as smoking contribute to GC risk [36]. Furthermore, diets high in salt, nitrites or smoked foods, pickled vegetables, and low in fruit and vegetable intake [23, 30, 37] are also thought to increase GC risk.

The influence of environmental factors on the genesis of GC is evident by the diminution of GC risk with migration from a higher incidence to lower incidence area [38]. Over the past several decades there has been a decline in the incidence of the IGC in the United States [39]. This echoes the worldwide decline in the overall incidence of GC, which has been attributed to alterations in diet, improved food storage and preservation, and decreased infection and colonization by *H. pylori*. The increased intake of fruits and vegetables combined with the advent of refrigeration has alleviated the need for food preservation by salt and other methods. Decreased crowding and improved living conditions are also felt to have reduced *H. pylori* exposure and as a result early colonization [40].

In contrast to the global decrease in GC incidence, the incidence of DGC, in particular the signet ring cell type, is not decreasing. Indeed, in North America, it may even be rising [39, 41]. The underlying cause for this increased incidence is not understood. *H. pylori* infection poses a similar risk for DGC as it does for IGC [42], although DGC is not linked to a precursor lesion. A prospective study examining baseline surrogate markers of *H. pylori* infection and chronic atrophic gastritis in patients who developed IGC or DGC showed an association between low titers of antibodies against *H. pylori* surface antigen in those that developed IGC and increased titers of antibodies in those that developed DGC. *H. pylori* only infects normal gastric mucosa, therefore these findings were consistent with expectations of decreased rates of *H. pylori* colonization in chronic atrophic gastritis, a known precursor to IGC [43]. There is evidence to support epigenetic effects of *H. pylori* infection, where promoter hypermethylation of *CDH1* in normal infected gastric mucosa was reversible with antibiotic treatment of the bacteria [44]. Furthermore methylation of *CDH1*, among other tumor suppressors, has been demonstrated in normal gastric mucosa of patients with GC, independent of the epigenetic modifications associated with normal aging [45]. In the context of particular *H. pylori* strains, individuals with a family history of GC had an increased risk of GC; however, due to the relatively small number of cases, there were no conclusions based on histological classifications [46]. Although there is no evidence of increased rates of *H. pylori* infection associated with the microscopic DGCs in the prophylactic gastrectomy specimens of *CDH1* mutation carriers, in light of its known role in GC carcinogenesis and in particular with regard to its ability to induce promoter hypermethylation of *CDH1*, *H. pylori* infection should be ruled out or treated in all *CDH1* mutation carriers.

1.3 Clinical Features of Gastric Cancer

Despite its low incidence in North America (~10 per 100,000 men and women per year), GC still remains a major health burden. According to the National Cancer Institute's Surveillance Epidemiology and End Results database, the overall 5-year relative survival rate for invasive GC from 1996 to 2004 was 24.7% (http://seer.cancer.gov/). For the most part, the poor survival rates are indicative of the delay in diagnoses. Early GC is usually clinically silent. Occasionally, it can present with gastrointestinal symptoms such as epigastric pain, dyspepsia, a sensation of gastric fullness, or frank symptoms of gastric obstruction. More often, GC is only detected following constitutional symptoms such as loss of weight. By then, the GC has usually progressed to stage III or locally invasive cancer. In countries where the incidences of GC are very high, nationwide screening programs utilize upper endoscopy as a means of detecting asymptomatic early-stage GC amenable to treatment by endoscopic resection. In Japan, this type of screening has proven effective at reducing GC-mortality rates [47]. However, in low-incidence countries, such as the United States, population-based endoscopic screening has not been implemented [48], because the incidence is too low to justify such an invasive screening program.

1.4 Overview of the Molecular Genetics of Gastric Cancer

Global genome analysis of GC by array comparative genomic hybridization has revealed recurrent regions of somatic copy number aberrations (CNAs). Frequent gains have been detected at 20q13, 8q24, and 7p [49–52] and frequent losses at 18q21, 3p14, 17p [48, 49, 51]. By correlating CNA with expression data, Tsukamoto et al. identified 114 genes significantly overexpressed in 14 amplified regions and 11 genes down-regulated in five deleted regions [49]. This data correlated overexpression of *DDX27, ARFGEF2, C20orf199, Kua-UEV, PTPN1, PARD6B, ADNP,* and *DPM1* with 20q13 amplification, which was present in 97% of the cases [49]. Deletion of 3p correlated with decreased expression of the putative tumor suppressor, *FHIT* [49], where abnormal sequence transcripts have been detected in a GC cell line [53] and decreased protein expression of FHIT has been found to correlate with undifferentiated tumors, diffuse histology, and poor prognosis [54]. Overexpression of genes occurs at many other amplified regions in particular *ERBB2* at 17q21 and *EGFR* at 7p11. *ERBB2* overexpression has been correlated with IGC and has been found to be significantly increased in metastatic disease [55] and to correlate with poor prognosis [56]. *EGFR* expression has also been associated with IGC where expression in the primary GC was shown to independently predict poor prognosis regardless of the expression level in the metastasis [55]. Deleted regions were also concordant with down-regulation of candidate tumor suppressors; *SMAD4* at 18q21 and *CDKN2B* at 9p21 [49]. Normal gastric mucosa, intestinal, and diffuse GC have been shown to have distinct cytogenetic profiles [57]. A consistent gain at 12q was reported in laser microdissected DGC ($n = 14$) and laser microdissected signet ring cell GC ($n = 7$) [49, 52].

1.4.1 The Tumor Suppressor p53

Mutations in *TP53*, which encodes the cell cycle control protein, p53, are common to many cancers. Over 950 different *TP53* mutations have been reported in stomach cancer (http://www-p53.iarc.fr/, R13, November 2008) [58]. The majority of mutations cause missense changes and occur between exons 5 and 8 which encode the DNA binding domain of the protein [59]. Mutations in *TP53* are preferentially associated with IGC rather than DGC. In a series of 62 GC, 17 out of 50 (34%) IGC had associated *TP53* mutations as compared with 0 out of 12 cases of DGC [60]. Incidentally, both IGC and DGC can occur in association with germline *TP53* mutations, which give rise to the familial cancer syndrome, Li–Fraumeni syndrome, where individuals are predisposed to an array of primary cancers. The genetic risks of the non-synonymous arginine/proline polymorphism at residue 72 of *TP53* have also been examined. The proline allele confers a reduced apoptotic ability and increased risk of cancer to the individual [61]. Additionally, in individuals with advanced GC, the proline genotype was associated with a lower response rate to chemotherapy [62].

1.4.2 Mismatch Repair Genes

Approximately 15% sporadic GCs exhibit microsatellite instability (MSI) [63]. This is due to genetic or epigenetic perturbations of the mismatch repair genes, *MLH1* or *MSH2* [64]. MSI probably functions in tumor progression rather than tumor initiation. This is supported by the finding of decreased hMLH1 protein expression and *MLH1* promoter hypermethylation in sporadic gastric carcinoma lesions with high MSI, but not in adjacent precursor lesions [65]. GC with high MSI tends to mainly occur in the antrum, be of the intestinal type, exhibits a predominantly lymphocytic infiltrate, occurs in the elderly, and has better survival rates with low metastatic rates [64–66]. Particular genes are frequently mutated in association with the defect in mismatch repair. There is high frequency of frameshift mutations found in the poly(A) tract of *TGFBR2*, the gene encoding a receptor for transforming growth factor β [66]. There is no apparent correlation with *TP53* mutations [60]. A recent comparison of the expression profiles of GCs with MSI and GCs without MSI revealed differential expression of genes involved in immune response, apoptotic pathways, and DNA repair pathways [60, 63]. This study and previous studies provide supportive evidence suggesting that the heightened immune response contributes to the longer survival rates.

Lynch syndrome [OMIM #120435], which is associated with germline mutations in the mismatch repair genes, leads to the development of colorectal and other cancers with MSI [67]. GC risk in the context of Lynch syndrome will be discussed below.

1.4.3 E-Cadherin

Decreased E-cadherin expression is a feature of many poorly differentiated epithelial cancers [68–71]. In particular, E-cadherin expression is down-regulated in sporadic DGC [68]. As highlighted above, molecular genetic differences exist between IGC and DGC; however overall, loss of E-cadherin expression remains the major discriminator between the two subtypes.

2 The Molecular Biology of *CDH1* and the Putative Role of E-Cadherin in Cancer

2.1 *Structure and Function of E-Cadherin*

E-cadherin belongs to a large family of transmembrane glycoproteins and is the primary mediator of epithelial cell–cell adhesion [72]. It has multiple roles in morphogenesis, cell polarization, structural organization of tissues [73], and cell migration [74], and is essential for normal development. Mouse embryos deficient in the protein fail to form a trophectodermal epithelium or a blastocyst [75]. *CDH1* [OMIM *192090] is located on chromosome 16q22.1. The genomic sequence of *CDH1* spans almost 100 kb and encodes 16 exons [76]. These 16 exons are transcribed and translated into the precursor protein which is cleaved prior to the delivery of molecules to the cell membrane as mature E-cadherin [77]. The mature E-cadherin protein contains three major domains: the extracellular domain encoded by exons 4–13, the transmembrane domain encoded by part of exon 13 and part of exon 14, and the highly conserved cytoplasmic domain encoded by the remainder of exon 14 to exon 16 [78]. E-cadherin is located at the basolateral surfaces of the epithelial cell where it forms dimers [79]. There, the large extracellular domain of E-cadherin, comprised of five cadherin repeats, homodimerizes with E-cadherin expressed on a neighboring epithelial cells in a Ca^{2+}-dependent manner, mediating cell–cell adhesion at the zonula adherens junctions. The cytosolic, carboxy-terminus of E-cadherin binds to β-catenin and α-catenin which in turn binds to the F-actin microfilaments of the cytoskeleton via α-catenin [72].

Several molecules have been implicated in the regulation of membrane trafficking of E-cadherin. p120-catenin, located at the juxtamembrane domain, not only strengthens the adhesion between cells but also plays a role in maintenance of E-cadherin at the membrane and degradation of the adhesion molecule [80, 81]. The members of the Rho family of GTPases contribute to epithelial morphogenesis, maintenance, adhesion, and cell migration in part through the regulation of E-cadherin and their downstream effects on the organization of the actin cytoskeleton [82–84].

The expression of E-cadherin is subject to positive and negative transcriptional regulation. Transcriptional repressors, such as Snail, Slug, dEF1/ZEB-1, Sip-1/ZEB-2, Twist, and E12/E47, bind to the E-box motifs at the *CDH1* promoter [85, 86]. Other regulatory regions outside of the promoter have also been identified such as the enhancer element in intron 2 [87]. In *CDH1*, intron 2 accounts for the majority of non-coding intronic sequence (~60 kb) and contains conserved *cis*-regulatory elements. The importance of intron 2 for normal expression of the gene has been underlined by a study of murine embryonic development following deletion of the intron in early mouse embryogenesis [85].

2.2 Variations in *CDH1* and the Association with Cancer

A *CDH1* promoter polymorphism at −160 C/A has been shown in vitro to have a role in transcriptional regulation, where the A allele was shown to have decreased transcriptional efficiency and weaker transcription factor binding affinity [88]. Analysis of eight *CDH1* haplotype-tagging polymorphisms, within the European Prospective Investigation into Cancer and Nutrition (EPIC-EURGAST) study, failed to demonstrate an elevated risk for GC for seven of the individual SNPs, including the

–160C/A polymorphism, or their associated haplotypes [89]. Likewise, no association was seen between the promoter polymorphism and GC risk in a recent Italian study [90]. However, meta-analysis ethnically stratifying cases and controls revealed the –160A allele to be a risk factor for GC in Europeans but not Asians [91]. As separate disease haplotypes in different populations could account for these discrepancies, it has been proposed that the positive associations could potentially be clinically relevant to the populations in which they were studied [92].

Recently another polymorphism in intron 2 was also associated with sporadic DGC in an Italian population [93]. This result will require validation in further studies.

The HDGC-associated germline *CDH1* mutations are dispersed across the gene [94] (Fig. 3.2). These mutations interfere with normal E-cadherin function in a variety of ways from alterations to conserved amino acid residues with predicted effects on protein structure, to deletions of critical domains, to protein truncation and haploinsufficiency due to nonsense-mediated mRNA decay. Recently our group reported large deletions as another genetic aberration of *CDH1* associated with 3.8% HDGC families [95].

Haploinsufficiency for E-cadherin is sufficient for normal development. However, there have been two families reported in which the inheritance of splicing

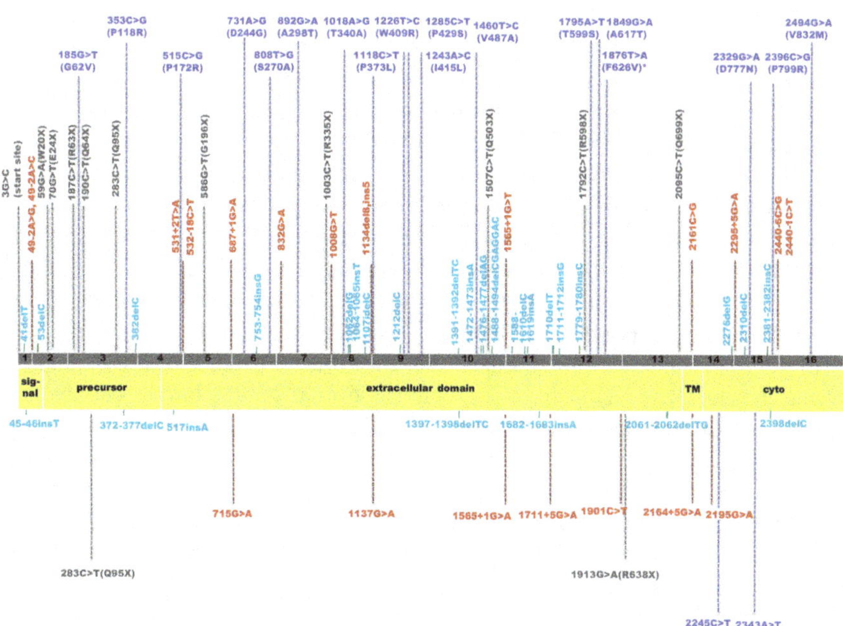

Fig. 3.2 Colors denote type of mutation (*light blue*: insertion/deletion; *brown*: splice site; *grey*: truncating; *dark blue*: missense). Mutations below *CDH1* occur in families with LBC history. Mutation marked with (*) indicates breast cancer history but not LBC

mutations in regions encoding the extracellular domain of E-cadherin (intron four splicing donor site; c.531+2 T>A and exon 8; c.1137G>A) has been associated with cleft lip with or without cleft palate [96]. Both mutations led to aberrant splicing which created in-frame deletions predicted to escape nonsense-mediated mRNA decay. Nonsense-mediated mRNA decay is the degradation of mRNA molecules containing a premature stop codon greater than 50 nucleotides prior to the last splice junction [97]. The abnormal splicing created by this mutation would result in a protein lacking parts of its extracellular cadherin binding domains. As E-cadherin is expressed in the frontonasal prominence, and the lateral and medial nasal prominences during the critical stages of lip and palate development [96], the authors postulated that the aberrant E-cadherin proteins might exert a dominant-negative effect over the wild-type E-cadherin protein by abnormal homodimerization. This association with cleft lip +/– cleft palate, however, was not seen in two other families with the c.1137G>A mutation [2], suggesting that the previous observation could have been due to a gene–environment interaction.

2.3 Loss of E-Cadherin and Cancer

The role of *CDH1* in cancer is believed to be related to the promotion of invasiveness caused by the loss of E-cadherin expression [98]. Cells deficient in E-cadherin lose the ability to adhere to each other and therefore become more invasive and metastasize [99]. The silencing of E-cadherin expression requires inactivation of both *CDH1* alleles either at the genetic level or at the epigenetic level. Intriguingly, re-expression of E-cadherin has been observed in the tumor cells at the metastatic site [100]. In sporadic DGC, the inactivation of the first allele is typically by mutations clustering in exons 8 and 9 resulting in exon-skipping and in-frame deletions of the extracellular domain [72]. Mutations and deletions in this critical area have been shown to have functional consequences [101]. Mutations in *CDH1* can be found in 50% of GC tumor specimens [102], where the inactivation of the remaining normal allele is often by hypermethylation of the *CDH1* promoter [103].

Loss of E-cadherin expression has been shown to be an early event as depicted by the in situ DGC lesion from a prophylactic total gastrectomy specimen of a *CDH1* mutation carrier shown in Fig. 3.3. Figure 3.3a is the H&E stain of the lesion and Fig. 3.3b shows the loss of membrane E-cadherin staining in the in situ signet ring cells indicating that the loss of E-cadherin is an early event which precedes invasion. Additionally, in sporadic LBC, in situ cancers situated beside their invasive counterparts also stain negatively for the cell adhesion molecule [104]; moreover they both share the same mutations in *CDH1* and harbor LOH of 16q [105], indicating that loss of E-cadherin is an early initiating event. The mechanism by which loss of E-cadherin protein expression occurs varies. E-cadherin expression can be heterogeneous depending on which part of the tumor is being tested. In addition to interpatient heterogeneity of the mechanisms that cause loss of expression of the normal allele of *CDH1*, there is also intrapatient heterogeneity whereby

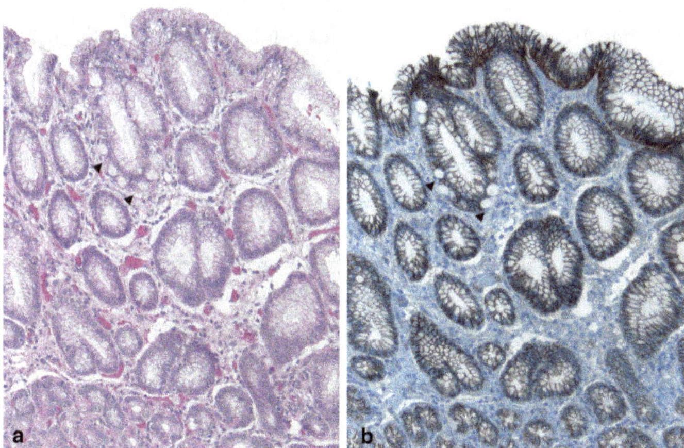

Fig. 3.3 These pictures show a small in situ focus of a diffuse gastric cancer from the same prophylactic gastrectomy specimen as shown in Fig. 3.1. (**a**) H&E stain. Note the similarity between the signet ring cells within the duct and the cross-section of a mucosal blood vessel; (**b**) E-cadherin stain showing down-regulated expression in the signet ring cells of the in situ focus of diffuse gastric cancer in comparison to the normal E-cadherin-positive epithelium. This picture implies that loss of E-cadherin expression is an early event in tumorigenesis. Photographs taken by Dr. Martin Köbel

different silencing mechanisms can be seen across and within patient's tumors [106]. Decreased expression of E-cadherin can also be a transient event, facilitating invasion and metastasis [107], with subsequent re-expression of E-cadherin in the metastatic cells [100]. Recently LOH was more frequently seen as the second hit in metastatic tumors [106].

The tumor suppressor function of E-cadherin [108–110] is supported by evidence of loss of expression of the other *CDH1* allele [106, 111, 112]. HDGC-associated GC exhibits a lack of expression of E-cadherin from the normal allele of *CDH1* that is achieved by epigenetic suppression of transcription or by mutation or loss of heterozygosity (LOH) [106, 111, 112]. LOH is a common phenomenon seen in association with loss of expression of tumor suppressor genes [113]. It refers to the somatic loss of the wild-type allele usually due to deletion of the gene or loss of a whole chromosome arm. It is detected by comparing microsatellite markers linked to the gene of interest in germline and tumor DNA. The markers in germline DNA are heterozygous, therefore the appearance of homozygosity in the markers of somatic tumor cells infers that there has been a loss of the wild-type allele [97].

The tumor suppressor role of E-cadherin is thought to be in part due to its association with β-catenin, a key player in the canonical Wnt signaling pathway [114]. The Wnt signaling pathway is implicated in familial adenomatous polyposis (FAP) where germline mutations in the *APC* [115] cause the autosomal dominant predisposition to gastrointestinal polyposis. Both β-catenin and APC are phosphorylated by the kinase, GSK3b resulting in ubiquitination and degradation of β-catenin.

Activation of the Wnt signaling cascade inhibits the activity of GSK3β. This causes an increase in the free cytoplasmic β-catenin molecule which then translocates to the nucleus and binds to the transcription factor, lymphocyte enhancer factor/T-cell factor (LEF1/Tcf). This results in transcription of Wnt responsive genes such as the oncogene, *c-Myc* [116, 117]. In addition to this role in regulating gene transcription, β-catenin also functions in epithelial cell adhesion through its association with E-cadherin and β-catenin. This association is thought to sequestrate β-catenin at the plasma membrane, thus preventing it from entering the nucleus. The existence of different forms of β-catenin with distinct binding properties has shed light on how the roles of β-catenin in cell adhesion and nuclear signaling might be regulated [118]. Thus, further elucidation of E-cadherin's relationship with this canonical oncogenic pathway is awaited.

3 Hereditary Gastric Cancer

3.1 The Crucial Role of Family History

Five to ten percent of GCs demonstrate familial clustering [119]. Shared environmental factors, such as diet and *H. pylori* infection, account for the majority of familial clustering of the intestinal type, although approximately 5% of the total GC burden is thought to be due to germline mutations in genes causing highly penetrant, autosomal dominant predispositions to cancer such as Lynch syndrome, Peutz–Jeghers syndrome (PJS), Li–Fraumeni syndrome (LFS), familial adenomatous polyposis (FAP), and HDGC [67].

Lynch syndrome or hereditary nonpolyposis colorectal cancer is caused by germline mutations in the mismatch repair genes: *hMSH2*, *hMLH1*, *hMSH6*, *hPMS1*, *hPMS2*. The syndrome is mainly characterized by susceptibility to colorectal cancer. However, after endometrial cancer, GC is the third most common cancer in these patients (in countries of low GC incidence). In a case series from the United Kingdom, GC accounted for 5% of cancers in families harboring *MLH1* or *MSH2* mutations [120].

IGC is the predominant subtype in Lynch syndrome [67]. The original Lynch syndrome family initially presented with a susceptibility to gastric and uterine cancer. However, over the years, the incidence of GC within this large pedigree has become insignificant compared to the incidence of cancer of the colon and endometrium [120]. This decrease in the incidence of GC in germline mutation carrying families largely echoes the overall decline in GC incidence in the general population. Although, in countries with higher incidences of GC, it is the second most common tumor associated with Lynch syndrome [122, 123].

With a relative risk of 213, GC is considered an integral tumor of the PJS caused by mutations in *STK11* [124].

LFS due to mutations in *TP53* or *CHEK2* is associated with both IGC and DGC [48, 125, 126].

FAP is caused by germline mutations in *APC*. GC occurs in 0.6% of patients [127]. A greater number of reports of GC (in particular IGC) associated with FAP have been reported in individuals from Japan, consistent with the overall higher incidences of sporadic GC in that population [128].

Increased risks of GC have also been found to be associated with *BRCA1* [128] and *BRCA2* mutation carriers [130, 131]. Reports of other genetic syndromes associated with GC exist although due to their paucity, it is hard to establish true associations.

Genome-wide association studies have uncovered low-to-moderate risk susceptibility genes for GC, although, currently, the clinical significance of these results is hard to interpret. Recently an intronic SNP in *PSCA*, encoding prostate stem cell antigen (PSCA), was identified in Japanese and Korean subjects, as having a significant association with DGC with an allele-specific odds ratio = 1.62, 95% CI, 1.39–1.89 [132]. Although the exact function of PSCA is not known, the protein is expressed in the normal gastric epithelium and lost in diffuse adenocarcinoma cells, indicating a possible tumor suppressor role in the gastric epithelium [132].

As previously mentioned the –160A/C promoter polymorphism of *CDH1* has also been investigated as increasing GC risk.

Until there is further understanding regarding the genetic variability among individuals who develop GC, the clinical interpretation of low-to-moderate penetrance genes associated with GC susceptibility will remain difficult. Even if validated, the relative risks associated with the –160A/C *CDH1* polymorphism and other germline polymorphisms such as in *PSCA*, are not high enough to be used to triage screening. Thus at this point, they do not appear clinically relevant [132].

Additionally, the interplay between environmental risk factors and the host's genetic background will also need to be considered. As previously eluded to, the polymorphisms; *IL-1B* -31T+, in the gene encoding IL-1β and *IL-1RN**2*2, in the gene encoding the receptor antagonist for IL-1β are thought to increase levels of IL-1β when the host is infected with *H. pylori*, leading to hypochlorhydria and increased GC [33]. The example of the IL-1β response to *H. pylori* infection highlights the importance of understanding gene–environment interactions to identify potentially modifiable risk factors such as *H. pylori* infection.

3.2 Hereditary Diffuse Gastric Cancer

The report of a Maori family with multiple cases of DGC inherited in a highly penetrant, autosomal dominant manner was first published in 1964 [133]. Three decades later this large family and two other Maori families with similar histories were analyzed using genetic linkage analysis to define a region on the long arm of chromosome 16 that included the *CDH1* locus [1]. Armed with this information and the knowledge of the role of somatic mutations of *CDH1* in sporadic GCs, Guilford identified *CDH1* germline truncating mutations in all three families [1]. This discovery has led to the subsequent identification of many more HDGC families of different ethnicities caused by novel or recurrent germline *CDH1* mutations or deletions [2, 3, 5, 6, 94, 96, 126, 134–149].

The International GC Linkage Consortium (IGCLC) was launched soon after the discovery of *CDH1* as a susceptibility gene for DGC. This created an international, multidisciplinary collaboration to develop a unified approach to the research and clinical management of the new syndrome, designated hereditary diffuse gastric cancer or HDGC [134]. The collective experience in testing over 160 probands from around the world has been that roughly half of these families can be accounted for by germline mutations or large deletions in *CDH1*. In families with HDGC, the risk for DGC appears to be independent of the common risk factors mentioned earlier.

Individuals harboring germline E-cadherin mutations have a lifetime risk of developing GC of 40–67% for males and a 63–83% for females [2, 3]. In both penetrance studies, females had a higher risk of developing GC [1, 2]. However, as we continue to extend family histories and find new HDGC families, recent unpublished data by the collaborative efforts of the IGCLC suggest that the risk for GC in males and females may be more similar than originally estimated (unpublished data). The average age of developing DGC is 38 years [78]; however, the range extends from 14 years of age up to 85 years of age [3]. The factors which determine the age of onset in a family remain to be elucidated. Thus, until it is understood what factors put people at higher risk for early-onset disease, appropriate screening should commence at least 5–10 years prior to the earliest reported diagnoses of cancer.

As of yet, no other genes have been associated with HDGC. Candidate gene studies in Portuguese families without *CDH1* mutations did not find germline mutations in *SMAD* or *caspase-10* [125]. Although they did identify a germline mutation in *TP53* in a family with multiple cases of GC, the histology of these cancers was not available [125]. Likewise there were no germline mutations in the candidate genes *RUNX3* and *HPP1* in German GC families [126]. Again, these investigators also found a germline *TP53* mutation in a 52-year-old proband with DGC and a family history of GC, leukemia (age 17), and hepatocellular carcinoma (age 34) in three first-degree relatives [126]. Germline *MET* mutations have also been found in two Korean probands with GC, the first had IGC with no age or family history specified, and the second occurred in a proband with DGC from a family selected based on the criteria of two first- or second-degree relatives affected with GC, at least one of whom was diagnosed with cancer before the age of 50 years [150]. Molecular testing for germline mutations in *MET* and other putative candidate genes such as *CTNNB1*, encoding β-catenin, in our *CDH1*-negative HDGC families has been negative (unpublished data). Even though mutations in *CDH1* may not be detected in all HDGC families, it has been shown that the majority of HDGC families display an imbalance of allele-specific *CDH1* expression, thus still implicating the locus in a proportion of *CDH1* mutation-negative HDGC families [151]. It is therefore possible that families with a compelling history of HDGC in whom coding mutations or deletions have not been identified, could have pathogenic mutations in regulatory or other non-coding regions of the *CDH1* gene [151].

3.3 Identification of At-Risk Individuals

The frequency with which *CDH1* germline mutations are detected in families with HDGC varies regionally, being higher in regions where there are low incidences of GC [2, 5, 6, 95, 125, 126]. In 1999 the definition of HDGC set forth by the IGCLC was any family meeting either of the following criteria: (1) two or more documented cases of DGC in first-/second-degree relatives, with at least one diagnosed under the age of 50 years or (2) three or more cases of documented DGC in first-/second-degree relatives, regardless of age of onset [78]. Using the initial selection criteria, the detection rates for germline mutations of *CDH1* have varied from as low as 11% [152] in high-incidence countries like Portugal to 30% in low-incidence areas such as North America [5]. To reflect the growing experience with HDGC, the updated IGCLC guidelines extend *CDH1* genetic testing to families with two cases of GC in which one case is histopathologically confirmed as DGC and diagnosed before the age of 50 (in submission). In addition, the guidelines endorse genetic testing of *CDH1* in families with both LBC and DGC, with one diagnosed before the age of 50, and in probands diagnosed with DGC before the age of 40, with no family history of GC [5, 6] (in submission). Recently we surveyed the incidence of *CDH1* aberrations in our HDGC families combined with HDGC families from different parts of the world that had either (1) three or more DGC in first-degree relatives diagnosed at any age or (2) two or more GC in first-degree relatives with at least one DGC diagnosed before age 50 years [95] and found that aberrations in *CDH1* occur in 46% of families. Keeping in mind that the majority of families came from areas of low gastric cancer incidence, this detection frequency likely overestimates the global contribution of *CDH1* mutations to HDGC families meeting these criteria, which likely lies around 25–30%.

4 Genetic Testing for *CDH1*

4.1 Genetic Counseling

Full screening of the *CDH1* gene is recommended in an individual fulfilling the HDGC criteria. DNA can generally be extracted from blood leukocytes, mucosal epithelial cells in saliva, or, with more difficulty and less accuracy, from normal tissue from paraffin blocks. Due to the problems with obtaining good quality DNA from paraffin blocks, an effort is always made to test DNA from living individuals. The decision to undergo genetic testing should only be made following adequate genetic counseling. There should be pre- and post-genetic testing counseling available which should provide the patient with information regarding HDGC, its mode of inheritance, and penetrance estimates of developing DGC and LBC. A discussion regarding the management options following a positive result (identification of a germline *CDH1* mutation or deletion) should be presented in the pre-genetic counseling appointment. Additionally, the patient should be made aware of the general risks and benefits of genetic testing.

The discussion of genetic testing should include ensuring that they understand the limitations of the analysis. While a negative result could indicate that the cancers in the family are unrelated to *CDH1*, it could also occur if a particular genetic abnormality of *CDH1* was not detected by the assay, resulting in a false-negative outcome. Thus, following a negative diagnostic test, cancer screening in the proband and blood-related family members should continue as before. Due to the uniqueness of each family's mutation, predictive testing can only become available to other members of the family at-risk once a mutation is found in an affected person or obligate carrier. Carrier testing of unaffected individuals allows for risk stratification and focusing of high-intensity screening in only those who are at risk.

In those who test negative for the family's mutation, the risk of DGC and LBC returns to that of the general population's and therefore screening for these individuals can be relaxed to population guidelines.

The psychosocial effects of genetic testing should be recognized, where some individuals may experience anxiety and distress relating to the results of the testing with regard to their personal and/or family risk of inherited cancer. This can potentially cause psychological distress in the individual and can affect family relationships.

As with most adult-onset genetic conditions, predictive testing is not generally offered to minors. However, as there are reports of individuals as young as 14 years of age being affected with DGC [1], with the consent of the parents or guardians and the appropriate consent from the minor, there are exceptions which can be made on a case-by-case basis. In this scenario, predictive testing would be used in order to determine if high-intensity surveillance would be necessary.

4.2 Methods of Testing

4.2.1 Mutation Screening

As germline *CDH1* mutations are heterozygous, various screening techniques designed to detect heterozygosity in the DNA have allowed targeted sequencing of exons displaying changes. Single strand conformation polymorphism (SSCP) rapidly detects single nucleotide substitutions in PCR amplicons by resolving differences in the electrophoretic mobility of the single-stranded amplicons [153]. The sensitivity of SSCP for mutation detection can be as high as 95% depending on the protocol [153]; however, SSCP requires highly stringent gel electrophoresis conditions.

Denaturing high-performance liquid chromatography (DHPLC) is an alternative method of mutation screening with improved sensitivity and capacity over SSCP. DHPLC detects heteroduplexes of the mutated and wild-type sequence upon partial denaturation and reannealing. The heteroduplexes are distinguished from the matched normal homoduplexes by their different melting temperatures on high-performance liquid chromatography. In both methods, exons in which sequence variations are detected are then bidirectionally sequenced to identify the heterozygous change. The popularity of these methods compared to direct sequencing of the gene was their lower cost. However, as sequencing costs are now a fraction of what they were 10 years ago, most laboratories have abandoned such techniques and use direct sequencing.

4.2.2 Sequencing

Currently in our laboratory, we screen for mutations of *CDH1* by bidirectionally sequencing the entire coding portion of *CDH1* including intron–exon boundaries [154]. The mutations range from small insertions and deletions to single base substitutions all of which can cause frameshifts or splicing abnormalities and lead to truncation of the protein or instability of the mRNA through nonsense-mediated mRNA decay. Truncating mutations are assumed to be pathogenic, whereas missense mutations that result in changes in an amino acid are harder to interpret in terms of their potential effect on E-cadherin's function, as distinguished from harmless variations in the gene. Computer software programs are used to predict the effect of a mutation on splicing and with regard to whether or not the amino acid change might affect the function of the protein. Although in general these predictions need to be validated by functional assays. Another test for pathogenic germline mutations in *CDH1* is that they should segregate with affected family members.

Functional characterization of a potentially pathogenic variant in *CDH1* is usually carried out by expression of a corresponding cDNA in a breast cancer cell line that does not usually express E-cadherin. The effect of expressing the E-cadherin with the variant amino acid in this cell line can then be compared with the effect of expressing the wild-type protein. E-cadherin function can then be assessed by assays studying proliferation rate, cell migration, cell aggregation, and cell invasiveness. Expression of the wild-type E-cadherin reverses the abnormalities in the E-cadherin negative breast cancer cell line, whereas expression of the mutated E-cadherin exhibits none or partial restoration of E-cadherin function. Pathogenic mutants of E-cadherin only partially reverse the defects in the breast cancer cell such as decreased cell aggregation and increased invasiveness.

A direct assessment of mutations potentially involved in splicing is by RNA analysis. If normal fresh frozen gastric tissue is not available for RNA extraction, *CDH1* is also expressed in leukocytes and mucosal epithelial cells of the mouth, therefore RNA extraction from blood or saliva samples is also possible. RT-PCR is performed on the patients RNA to create the coding DNA in order to determine if abnormal transcripts are present.

Minigene assays can also be used to determine splicing effects of a mutation. By creating an expression construct which harbors the exon with the mutation of interest surrounded by its neighboring introns and exons, the identification of unexpected transcripts indicates that the mutation alters normal splicing.

4.2.3 Large Deletion Analysis

Mutation-negative cases are subjected to multiplex ligation-dependent probe amplification (MLPA), a method which enables detection of copy number variation in genomic sequences. Using this technique, our group has identified large deletions in *CDH1* which segregate with disease in 6.5% of HDGC *CDH1* mutation-negative families [94]. Overall large deletions of *CDH1* account for approximately 4% of HDGC [94].

4.2.4 Testing Stratification

In Newfoundland, an island province located off of the east coast of Canada, we recently identified a founder mutation in several different branches of a large family [2]. In light of the isolated population and our discovery of four other mutations in different families of Newfoundland heritage, we currently test families of Newfoundland heritage using a stepwise approach, consisting of an initial screen for the panel of known mutations that have already been found in the province, prior to full *CDH1* sequencing.

5 Clinical Management

5.1 *Management for the Risk of Gastric Cancer*

Due to the highly penetrant nature of HDGC caused by mutations in *CDH1*, at-risk individuals should have annual surveillance endoscopy with multiple random biopsies, beginning in their early twenties [16, 67]. A detailed description of surveillance protocols can be found in the latest consensus guidelines from the IGCLC (in submission). The necessity for multiple biopsies is supported by the finding that increasing numbers of random biopsies taken on surveillance endoscopy positively correlate with detection of invasive foci of DGC [17]. The decision of when to start surveillance is based on the average age of DGC diagnosis being around 40 years, although there are families in which individuals as young as 14 years of age have been diagnosed [1]. Thus screening of at-risk individuals should generally begin 5–10 years prior to the earliest cancer diagnosis in the family. At-risk individuals are those who are known to carry mutations in *CDH1* or those who belong to HDGC families and *CDH1* mutation status is not known.

Several other screening modalities have been tested including chromoendoscopy [12], PET scan [155], endoscopic ultrasound, stool for guaiac, abdominal CT, and multiple random stomach biopsies [16]. Unfortunately these do not reliably detect DGC, as demonstrated by the finding of multiple small cancer foci in six out of six gastrectomy specimens from *CDH1* mutation carriers only a week following an unremarkable panel of these investigations [16]. Despite the inability of endoscopy to reliably detect very small cancer foci, it has a greater likelihood of identifying clinically relevant cancers of more advanced stage that are more likely to metastasize. Therefore regular surveillance by endoscopy with multiple random biopsies still remains an important alternative to gastrectomy [16] and should be strongly recommended in those delaying PTG or electing against it.

5.2 Prophylactic Total Gastrectomy

Prophylactic total gastrectomy (PTG) is recommended for *CDH1* germline mutation carriers. PTG is achieved by Roux-en-y esophagojejunostomy [16] with extreme caution as to obtaining adequate proximal margins to ensure all of the gastric mucosa has been removed. The chief argument for undertaking such a dramatic risk-reduction strategy is that multiple PTGs carried out in germline *CDH1* mutation carriers have retrospectively become curative surgeries upon the finding of multiple small foci of invasive DGC within the resected organs [7–19, 67].

PTG is a major operation where, beyond surgical complications such as anastomotic leakage, strictures, or septic complications, there is a virtually 100% morbidity rate for complications such as altered eating habits, loss of weight, and diarrhea [8]. In a young and healthy individual, the risk of mortality with total gastrectomy in an experienced surgeon's hands is estimated to be less than 1% [67]. These estimates are below those quoted in the literature (3.5%) which are based upon total gastrectomies performed with curative intent for clinical GC in an older patient demographic [156].

Management by a multidisciplinary team approach which includes a dietician, gastroenterologist, geneticist, and general surgeon is extremely important in order to counsel the patient adequately regarding the risks, benefits, and clinical sequelae of this major operation [157]. This surgery has a major impact on the patient's nutritional status and ability to maintain adequate caloric intake and maintain normal vitamin and mineral stores with appropriate supplementation. Thus ongoing follow-up with the multidisciplinary team to monitor and correct any abnormal nutritional parameters is essential. Expected deficiencies post-gastrectomy include vitamin B_{12} deficiency, due to the removal of the production source for intrinsic factor required to absorb the vitamin. There is also an expectation for the malabsorption of iron, calcium, folate and the fat soluble vitamins underscoring the importance of the involvement of a multidisciplinary team to monitor for this. The morbidity that can be expected post-gastrectomy usually worsens in the first 3–6 months post-gastrectomy but then gradually improves [16]. Due to the weight loss and nutritional implications, prophylactic gastrectomy is not generally recommended until the growth period is finished. However, this decision must also be weighed against the age of the youngest person in the family diagnosed with GC [7]. In families where there are cases of early-onset gastric cancer, prophylactic gastrectomy should be considered sooner on a case-by-case basis in combination with earlier commencement of regular endoscopic screening prior to surgery. In the past we have been hesitant to recommend gastrectomy in females prior to completion of childbearing; however, we have recently been acquiring encouraging evidence to suggest that women can successfully carry healthy pregnancies post-gastrectomy [158].

To date there have not been any reports of cancer in a member of an HDGC family post-prophylactic total gastrectomy.

6 Aberrations of *CDH1* and Lobular Breast Cancer

In addition to the high lifetime risk of GC, in females within HDGC families there is an increased lifetime risk of breast cancer (39–52%) [2, 3]. In HDGC families there is particular association with the lobular breast cancer (LBC). The average age of onset for breast cancer was found to be 53 years [3].

We have reported two novel germline *CDH1* mutations in a families with hereditary LBC and no known history of GC, and in one family in which LBC was the predominant cancer diagnosis [159, 160]. No genotype–phenotype relationships have been determined for the mutations seen in hereditary LBC or LBC-associated HDGC families, although a weakly statistically significant trend is apparent toward the 3′ end of the gene [160]. As breast cancers related to germline *CDH1* mutation carrier status correlate with the lobular subtype, the capacity exists to identify potential *CDH1* mutation carriers based on morphologic grounds. To date, our data show that non-synonymous *CDH1* variants may contribute only a small amount to individuals with a diagnosis of LBC selected based on a family history of breast cancer or young age of the proband at diagnosis (unpublished data). It is likely that improved detection rates will depend upon more stringent selection criteria such as multiple early-onset cases of LBC in first- or second-degree relatives or alternatively multiple cases of LBC in addition to a history of gastric cancer.

6.1 Epidemiology of LBC

In North America breast cancer (BC) is the most common cancer diagnosis in women where 1:9 women will develop the cancer in their lifetime. The majority of primary breast cancers are adenocarcinomas, where infiltrating ductal carcinoma (IDC) accounts for the majority of breast cancer diagnoses and LBC only comprises about 10% of cases. LBC characteristically has a loose, ill-defined architecture as compared with IDC [161]. Instead of forming discrete glandular structures, the malignant cells in LBC exhibit infiltrative behavior and dissociate from the ductal unit to become isolated and highly dispersive, invading the stroma in single files [104]. Signet ring cells analogous to those seen in DGC are also seen in LBC and like DGC, LBC characteristically stains negative for E-cadherin [162].

6.2 Sporadic Breast Cancer

In addition to its role in GC, E-cadherin also plays a similar role in LBC. There are striking similarities between the behavioral and morphologic phenotypes of both the DGC and the LBC. Both share features such as poor differentiation and a high mucin content giving rise to a signet ring appearance. Individual cancer cells are also non-cohesive, highly dispersive, and invasive. Thus sporadic LBC cells look and behave in a similar fashion to DGC where 86% stain negatively for E-cadherin [104]. Indeed, *CDH1* mutations can also be found in 56% of LBC tumor specimens [163]. In sporadic LBC, the majority of mutations are truncating [163], and the second hit is usually by loss of heterozygosity (LOH) or promoter methylation [163, 164].

6.3 Hereditary Breast Cancer

Hereditary breast cancer accounts for 5–10% of breast cancer cases where a significant proportion of cases are caused by germline *BRCA1* or *BRCA2* mutations [165]. Other breast cancer susceptibility genes include *TP53* (LFS), *PTEN* (Cowden syndrome), *ATM*, *BRIP1*, *PALB2*, and *CHEK2* [166, 167].

Germline *CDH1* mutations have been shown to have a role in hereditary lobular breast cancer. The potential association of LBC to HDGC was postulated soon after there appeared to be an increased incidence of breast cancer in the HDGC syndrome. This was on the basis of known *CDH1* aberrations in sporadic LBC [134]. Keller et al. initially described an LBC and a DGC in a *CDH1* mutation carrier [4]. Further supportive evidence came from the identification of further HDGC families in which there was an overrepresentation of the LBC subtype [5, 6]. The risk seems to be only for female breast cancer as there have not been any reports of male breast cancer associated with HDGC families. By screening for germline mutations of *CDH1* in LBC probands selected based on young age or family history of breast cancer, we confirmed the association of LBC with germline mutations of *CDH1* [159].

6.4 Lobular Breast Cancer Risk

6.4.1 Screening

Currently there is not enough data on women with germline *CDH1* mutations and the development of breast cancer to determine the best risk-reduction and breast cancer screening strategies. Thus, recommendations for LBC risk management for women who are known carriers of *CDH1* mutations or those that have an unknown mutation status are derived from the experiences with managing other highly penetrant familial breast cancer syndromes. In accordance with recommendations for screening other highly penetrant hereditary breast cancer syndromes, these women should have annual screening mammograms and breast MRI; perform breast self-examination and have semi-annual clinical breast examination starting at around age 30, or 5–10 years prior to the earliest breast cancer diagnosis in the family [160, 168]. The American Cancer Society recommends MRI in addition to mammography in women with a lifetime risk of breast cancer greater than 20–25% [169]. Thus, the 39–52% lifetime risk of breast cancer in women conferred by germline *CDH1* mutations [2, 3] well exceeds their minimum range. LBC is difficult to detect by mammography, thus the use of MRI in this hereditary cancer syndrome where there is a particular susceptibility to LBC is attractive. Furthermore, there is evidence to suggest some increased detection of LCIS [170].

6.4.2 Chemoprophylaxis

Most LBCs are estrogen-receptor positive [161], and as both tamoxifen and ralox-ifene have been shown to reduce the risk of estrogen-receptor positive [171, 172] breast cancers in randomized trials, this is a conceivable strategy for chemopre-vention [16], although at this time is unproven. Of theoretical benefit to *CDH1* mutation carriers is that the risk reduction with both agents was greatest in women with lobular carcinoma in situ [173].

6.4.3 Prophylactic Mastectomy

Prophylactic mastectomy has been very effective as a primary risk-reduction strat-egy in women with *BRCA1* or *BRCA2* mutations, reducing their risks up to 90% [174]. Prophylactic mastectomy may also be considered in *CDH1* mutation-positive women; however, at this time not enough data exist to recommend this as a primary risk-reduction strategy in *CDH1* mutation carriers. It would likely be a logical alter-native to those women who have previously undergone treatment for breast cancer in one breast or those who have withstood multiple false-positive biopsies requiring further confirmatory biopsies. Although prophylactic mastectomy can significantly decrease a woman's risk of developing breast cancer, women undergoing the pro-cedure are at risk of a range of physical complications and potential psychological sequelae thus necessitating full counseling prior to the woman making a decision regarding the surgery [175]. The counseling should include the risk of possible altered perception of the body and the sexual relationship and the possibility of a negative physical impact of surgery [176].

7 Screening for Risk of Other Cancers in *CDH1*

Although there have been reports of signet ring colon cancer in families with germline *CDH1* mutations [6, 94], currently there is not enough evidence to rec-ommend colon cancer screening in all HDGC families. In HDGC families in which there is an additional family history of colon cancer, in particular of the signet ring cell subtype, it would be prudent to undertake more intense colon cancer screening such as commencing screening by colonoscopy every 3–5 years beginning at age 40 years or 10 years younger than the youngest colon cancer (which ever is younger) (IGCLC guidelines, in submission). Thus, at this stage these families should be judged on a case-by-case basis.

Whether germline *CDH1* mutation carriers are at higher risk of other cancers still remains to be elucidated. Various other cancers have been reported in isolated families [2, 149]. Prostate cancer has been reported in a germline *CDH1* mutation carrier [135], and the −160 C/A *CDH1* polymorphism has also been implicated in association with the disease in Europeans and Asians [177]; however, currently, there is no conclusive association with this or other cancers.

8 Concluding Thoughts

Since the causative gene for HDGC has been identified, PTG has emerged as the primary risk-reduction strategy. Future studies are necessary to determine the long-term sequelae of PTG including quality of life issues and establishing what other potential cancers *CDH1* mutation carriers will now be at risk of. The almost complete penetrance for multifocal disease found in PTG specimens following exhaustive review mandates further study of the biology behind what causes some of the minute foci of invasive cancer to progress to clinically relevant disease. This will require a better understanding of tumor progression in mutation carriers and the host and environmental risk factors which contribute to this. Understanding the biological basis for disease progression will enable us to develop improved methods of surveillance for cancer progression, which could obviate the need for such radical risk-reduction surgeries and may also lead to new pharmacologic prophylactic measures.

References

1. Guilford P, Hopkins J, Harraway J et al (1998) E-cadherin germline mutations in familial gastric cancer. Nature 392:402–405
2. Kaurah P, MacMillan A, Boyd N et al (2007) Founder and recurrent CDH1 mutations in families with hereditary diffuse gastric cancer. JAMA 297:2360–2372
3. Pharoah PD, Guilford P, Caldas C, International Gastric Cancer Linkage Consortium (2001) Incidence of gastric cancer and breast cancer in CDH1 (E-cadherin) mutation carriers from hereditary diffuse gastric cancer families. Gastroenterology 121:1348–1353
4. Keller G, Vogelsang H, Becker I et al (1999) Diffuse type gastric and lobular breast carcinoma in a familial gastric cancer patient with an E-cadherin germline mutation. Am J Pathol 155:337–342
5. Suriano G, Yew S, Ferreira P et al (2005) Characterization of a recurrent germ line mutation of the E-cadherin gene: implications for genetic testing and clinical management. Clin Cancer Res 11:5401–5409
6. Brooks-Wilson AR, Kaurah P, Suriano G et al (2004) Germline E-cadherin mutations in hereditary diffuse gastric cancer: assessment of 42 new families and review of genetic screening criteria. J Med Genet 41:508–517
7. Huntsman DG, Carneiro F, Lewis FR et al (2001) Early gastric cancer in young, asymptomatic carriers of germ-line E-cadherin mutations. N Engl J Med 344:1904–1909
8. Lewis FR, Mellinger JD, Hayashi A et al (2001) Prophylactic total gastrectomy for familial gastric cancer. Surgery 130:612–617, discussion 617–619

9. Chun YS, Lindor NM, Smyrk TC et al (2001) Germline E-cadherin gene mutations: is prophylactic total gastrectomy indicated? Cancer 92:181–187
10. Carneiro F, Huntsman DG, Smyrk TC et al (2004) Model of the early development of diffuse gastric cancer in E-cadherin mutation carriers and its implications for patient screening. J Pathol 203:681–687
11. Charlton A, Blair V, Shaw D, Parry S, Guilford P, Martin IG (2004) Hereditary diffuse gastric cancer: predominance of multiple foci of signet ring cell carcinoma in distal stomach and transitional zone. Gut 53:814–820
12. Shaw D, Blair V, Framp A et al (2005) Chromoendoscopic surveillance in hereditary diffuse gastric cancer: an alternative to prophylactic gastrectomy? Gut 54:461–468
13. Gaya DR, Stuart RC, McKee RF, Going JJ, Davidson R, Stanley AJ (2005) E-cadherin mutation-associated diffuse gastric adenocarcinoma: penetrance and non-penetrance. Eur J Gastroenterol Hepatol 17:1425–1428
14. Blair V, Martin I, Shaw D et al (2006) Hereditary diffuse gastric cancer: diagnosis and management. Clin Gastroenterol Hepatol 4:262–275
15. Francis WP, Rodrigues DM, Perez NE, Lonardo F, Weaver D, Webber JD (2007) Prophylactic laparoscopic-assisted total gastrectomy for hereditary diffuse gastric cancer. JSLS 11:142–147
16. Norton JA, Ham CM, Van Dam J et al (2007) CDH1 truncating mutations in the E-cadherin gene: an indication for total gastrectomy to treat hereditary diffuse gastric cancer. Ann Surg 245:873–879
17. Barber ME, Save V, Carneiro F et al (2008) Histopathological and molecular analysis of gastrectomy specimens from hereditary diffuse gastric cancer patients has implications for endoscopic surveillance of individuals at risk. J Pathol 216:286–294
18. Rogers WM, Dobo E, Norton JA et al (2008) Risk-reducing total gastrectomy for germline mutations in E-cadherin (CDH1): pathologic findings with clinical implications. Am J Surg Pathol 32:799–809
19. Hebbard PC, Macmillan A, Huntsman D et al (2009) Prophylactic total gastrectomy (PTG) for hereditary diffuse gastric cancer (HDGC): the Newfoundland experience with 23 patients. Ann Surg Oncol 16:1890–1895
20. LAUREN P (1965) The two histological main types of gastric carcinoma: diffuse and so-called intestinal-type carcinoma. an attempt at a histo-clinical classification. Acta Pathol Microbiol Scand 64:31–49
21. Crew KD, Neugut AI (2006) Epidemiology of gastric cancer. World J Gastroenterol 12: 354–362
22. Correa P (1992) Human gastric carcinogenesis: a multistep and multifactorial process – first American cancer society award lecture on cancer epidemiology and prevention. Cancer Res 52:6735–6740
23. Oliveira C, Moreira H, Seruca R et al (2005) Role of pathology in the identification of hereditary diffuse gastric cancer: Report of a Portuguese family. Virchows Arch 446: 181–184
24. Humar B, Fukuzawa R, Blair V et al (2007) Destabilized adhesion in the gastric proliferative zone and c-src kinase activation mark the development of early diffuse gastric cancer. Cancer Res 67:2480–2489
25. Hamilton SR, Aaltonen LA (2000) Pathology and genetics. Tumours of the digestive system, WHO classification of tumours, vol 2. IARC Press, France, pp 35–52
26. Parkin DM, Bray F, Ferlay J, Pisani P (2005) Global cancer statistics, 2002. CA Cancer J Clin 55:74–108
27. Suerbaum S, Michetti P (2002) Helicobacter pylori infection. N Engl J Med 347: 1175–1186
28. Uemura N, Okamoto S, Yamamoto S et al (2001) Helicobacter pylori infection and the development of gastric cancer. N Engl J Med 345:784–789

29. Helicobacter and Cancer Collaborative Group (2001) Gastric cancer and helicobacter pylori: a combined analysis of 12 case control studies nested within prospective cohorts. Gut 49:347–353

30. Ferreira AC, Isomoto H, Moriyama M, Fujioka T, Machado JC, Yamaoka Y (2008) Helicobacter and gastric malignancies. Helicobacter 13(Supplement 1):28–34

31. Stein M, Rappuoli R, Covacci A (2000) Tyrosine phosphorylation of the helicobacter pylori CagA antigen after cag-driven host cell translocation. Proc Natl Acad Sci U S A 97: 1263–1268

32. Ohnishi N, Yuasa H, Tanaka S et al (2008) Transgenic expression of helicobacter pylori CagA induces gastrointestinal and hematopoietic neoplasms in mouse. Proc Natl Acad Sci U S A 105:1003–1008

33. El-Omar EM, Carrington M, Chow WH et al (2000) Interleukin-1 polymorphisms associated with increased risk of gastric cancer. Nature 404:398–402

34. El-Omar EM, Rabkin CS, Gammon MD et al (2003) Increased risk of noncardia gastric cancer associated with proinflammatory cytokine gene polymorphisms. Gastroenterology 124:1193–1201

35. Canedo P, Corso G, Pereira F et al (2008) The interferon gamma receptor 1 (IFNGR1) – 56C/T gene polymorphism is associated with increased risk of early gastric carcinoma. Gut 57:1504–1508

36. Forman D, Burley VJ (2006) Gastric cancer: global pattern of the disease and an overview of environmental risk factors. Best Pract Res Clin Gastroenterol 20:633–649

37. Liu C, Russell RM (2008) Nutrition and gastric cancer risk: an update. Nutr Rev 66:237–249

38. McMichael AJ, McCall MG, Hartshorne JM, Woodings TL (1980) Patterns of gastro-intestinal cancer in European migrants to Australia: the role of dietary change. Int J Cancer 25:431–437

39. Henson DE, Dittus C, Younes M, Nguyen H, Albores-Saavedra J (2004) Differential trends in the intestinal and diffuse types of gastric carcinoma in the united states, 1973–2000: increase in the signet ring cell type. Arch Pathol Lab Med 128:765–770

40. Roosendaal R, Kuipers EJ, Buitenwerf J et al (1997) Helicobacter pylori and the birth cohort effect: evidence of a continuous decrease of infection rates in childhood. Am J Gastroenterol 92:1480–1482

41. Borch K, Jonsson B, Tarpila E et al (2000) Changing pattern of histological type, location, stage and outcome of surgical treatment of gastric carcinoma. Br J Surg 87:618–626

42. Kamangar F, Dawsey SM, Blaser MJ et al (2006) Opposing risks of gastric cardia and noncardia gastric adenocarcinomas associated with helicobacter pylori seropositivity. J Natl Cancer Inst 98:1445–1452

43. Tatemichi M, Sasazuki S, Inoue M, Tsugane S, Japan Public Health Center Study Group (2008) Different etiological role of helicobacter pylori (hp) infection in carcinogenesis between differentiated and undifferentiated gastric cancers: a nested case-control study using IgG titer against hp surface antigen. Acta Oncol 47:360–365

44. Perri F, Cotugno R, Piepoli A et al (2007) Aberrant DNA methylation in non-neoplastic gastric mucosa of H. pylori infected patients and effect of eradication. Am J Gastroenterol 102:1361–1371

45. Kaise M, Yamasaki T, Yonezawa J, Miwa J, Ohta Y, Tajiri H (2008) CpG island hyperme-thylation of tumor-suppressor genes in H. pylori-infected non-neoplastic gastric mucosa is linked with gastric cancer risk. Helicobacter 13:35–41

46. Brenner H, Arndt V, Sturmer T, Stegmaier C, Ziegler H, Dhom G (2000) Individual and joint contribution of family history and helicobacter pylori infection to the risk of gastric carcinoma. Cancer 88:274–279

47. Lee KJ, Inoue M, Otani T et al (2006) Gastric cancer screening and subsequent risk of gastric cancer: a large-scale population-based cohort study, with a 13-year follow-up in Japan. Int J Cancer 118:2315–2321

48. Sugano K (2008) Gastric cancer: pathogenesis, screening, and treatment. Gastrointest Endosc Clin N Am 18:513–522
49. Tsukamoto Y, Uchida T, Karnan S et al (2008) Genome-wide analysis of DNA copy number alterations and gene expression in gastric cancer. J Pathol 216:471–482
50. Wang LD, Qin YR, Fan ZM et al (2006) Comparative genomic hybridization: comparison between esophageal squamous cell carcinoma and gastric cardia adenocarcinoma from a high-incidence area for both cancers in Henan, northern china. Dis Esophagus 19:459–467
51. Kang JU, Kang JJ, Kwon KC et al (2006) Genetic alterations in primary gastric carcinomas correlated with clinicopathological variables by array comparative genomic hybridization. J Korean Med Sci 21:656–665
52. Kurihara Y, Ghazizadeh M, Bo H et al (2002) Genome-wide screening of laser capture microdissected gastric signet ring cell carcinomas. J Nippon Med Sch 69:235–242
53. Lee SH, Kim HS (2003) Sequence analyses of aberrant FHIT transcripts in gastric cancer cell lines. Korean J Gastroenterol 42:476–483
54. Rocco A, Schandl L, Chen J et al (2003) Loss of FHIT protein expression correlates with disease progression and poor differentiation in gastric cancer. J Cancer Res Clin Oncol 129:84–88
55. Kim JH, Kim MA, Lee HS, Kim WH (2009) Comparative analysis of protein expressions in primary and metastatic gastric carcinomas. Hum Pathol 40:314–322
56. Barros-Silva JD, Leitao D, Afonso L et al (2009) Association of ERBB2 gene status with histopathological parameters and disease-specific survival in gastric carcinoma patients. Br J Cancer 100:487–493
57. Myllykangas S, Junnila S, Kokkola A et al (2008) Integrated gene copy number and expression microarray analysis of gastric cancer highlights potential target genes. Int J Cancer 123:817–825
58. Petitjean A, Mathe E, Kato S et al (2007) Impact of mutant p53 functional properties on TP53 mutation patterns and tumor phenotype: lessons from recent developments in the IARC TP53 database. Hum Mutat 28:622–629
59. Petitjean A, Achatz MI, Borresen-Dale AL, Hainaut P, Olivier M (2007) TP53 mutations in human cancers: functional selection and impact on cancer prognosis and outcomes. Oncogene 26:2157–2165
60. Migliavacca M, Ottini L, Bazan V et al (2004) TP53 in gastric cancer: mutations in the l3 loop and LSH motif DNA-binding domains of TP53 predict poor outcome. J Cell Physiol 200:476–485
61. Imyanitov EN (2009) Gene polymorphisms, apoptotic capacity and cancer risk. Hum Genet 125:239–246
62. Kim JG, Sohn SK, Chae YS et al (2008) TP53 codon 72 polymorphism associated with prognosis in patients with advanced gastric cancer treated with paclitaxel and cisplatin. Cancer Chemother Pharmacol 64(2):355–360
63. D'Errico M, de Rinaldis E, Blasi MF et al (2009) Genome-wide expression profile of sporadic gastric cancers with microsatellite instability. Eur J Cancer 45:461–469
64. Falchetti M, Saieva C, Lupi R et al (2008) Gastric cancer with high-level microsatellite instability: target gene mutations, clinicopathologic features, and long-term survival. Hum Pathol 39:925–932
65. Leung SY, Yuen ST, Chung LP, Chu KM, Chan AS, Ho JC (1999) hMLH1 promoter methylation and lack of hMLH1 expression in sporadic gastric carcinomas with high-frequency microsatellite instability. Cancer Res 59:159–164
66. Wu MS, Lee CW, Shun CT et al (2000) Distinct clinicopathologic and genetic profiles in sporadic gastric cancer with different mutator phenotypes. Genes Chromosomes Cancer 27:403–411
67. Lynch HT, Grady W, Suriano G, Huntsman D (2005) Gastric cancer: new genetic developments. J Surg Oncol 90:114–133, discussion 133

68. Mayer B, Johnson JP, Leitl F et al (1993) E-cadherin expression in primary and metastatic gastric cancer: down-regulation correlates with cellular dedifferentiation and glandular disintegration. Cancer Res 53:1690–1695

69. Gamallo C, Palacios J, Suarez A et al (1993) Correlation of E-cadherin expression with differentiation grade and histological type in breast carcinoma. Am J Pathol 142:987–993

70. Kadowaki T, Shiozaki H, Inoue M et al (1994) E-cadherin and alpha-catenin expression in human esophageal cancer. Cancer Res 54:291–296

71. Winter JM, Ting AH, Vilardell F et al (2008) Absence of E-cadherin expression distinguishes noncohesive from cohesive pancreatic cancer. Clin Cancer Res 14:412–418

72. Berx G, Becker KF, Hofler H, van Roy F (1998) Mutations of the human E-cadherin (CDH1) gene. Hum Mutat 12:226–237

73. Keller R (2002) Shaping the vertebrate body plan by polarized embryonic cell movements. Science 298:1950–1954

74. Geisbrecht ER, Montell DJ (2002) Myosin VI is required for E-cadherin-mediated border cell migration. Nat Cell Biol 4:616–620

75. Larue L, Ohsugi M, Hirchenhain J, Kemler R (1994) E-cadherin null mutant embryos fail to form a trophectoderm epithelium. Proc Natl Acad Sci U S A 91:8263–8267

76. Berx G, Staes K, van Hengel J et al (1995) Cloning and characterization of the human invasion suppressor gene E-cadherin (CDH1). Genomics 26:281–289

77. Shore EM, Nelson WJ (1991) Biosynthesis of the cell adhesion molecule uvomorulin (E-cadherin) in Madin-Darby canine kidney epithelial cells. J Biol Chem 266:19672–19680

78. Caldas C, Carneiro F, Lynch HT et al (1999) Familial gastric cancer: overview and guidelines for management. J Med Genet 36:873–880

79. Boller K, Vestweber D, Kemler R (1985) Cell-adhesion molecule uvomorulin is localized in the intermediate junctions of adult intestinal epithelial cells. J Cell Biol 100:327–332

80. Thoreson MA, Anastasiadis PZ, Daniel JM et al (2000) Selective uncoupling of p120(ctn) from E-cadherin disrupts strong adhesion. J Cell Biol 148:189–202

81. Xiao K, Oas RG, Chiasson CM, Kowalczyk AP (2007) Role of p120-catenin in cadherin trafficking. Biochim Biophys Acta 1773:8–16

82. Van Aelst L, Symons M (2002) Role of rho family GTPases in epithelial morphogenesis. Genes Dev 16:1032–1054

83. Fujita Y, Hogan C, Braga VM (2006) Regulation of cell-cell adhesion by Rap1. Methods Enzymol 407:359–372

84. Shen Y, Hirsch DS, Sasiela CA, Wu WJ (2008) Cdc42 regulates E-cadherin ubiquitination and degradation through an epidermal growth factor receptor to src-mediated pathway. J Biol Chem 283:5127–5137

85. Stemmler MP, Hecht A, Kemler R (2005) E-cadherin intron 2 contains cis-regulatory elements essential for gene expression. Development 132:965–976

86. Gloushankova NA (2008) Changes in regulation of cell-cell adhesion during tumor transformation. Biochemistry (Mosc) 73:742–750

87. Sorkin BC, Jones FS, Cunningham BA, Edelman GM (1993) Identification of the promoter and a transcriptional enhancer of the gene encoding L-CAM, a calcium-dependent cell adhesion molecule. Proc Natl Acad Sci U S A 90:11356–11360

88. Li LC, Chui RM, Sasaki M et al (2000) A single nucleotide polymorphism in the E-cadherin gene promoter alters transcriptional activities. Cancer Res 60:873–876

89. Jenab M, McKay JD, Ferrari P et al (2008) CDH1 gene polymorphisms, smoking, helicobacter pylori infection and the risk of gastric cancer in the European prospective investigation into cancer and nutrition (EPIC-EURGAST). Eur J Cancer 44:774–780

90. Corso G, Berardi A, Marrelli D et al (2009) CDH1 C-160A promoter polymorphism and gastric cancer risk. Eur J Cancer Prev 18:46–49

91. Wang GY, Lu CQ, Zhang RM, Hu XH, Luo ZW (2008) The E-cadherin gene polymorphism 160C–>A and cancer risk: a HuGE review and meta-analysis of 26 case-control studies. Am J Epidemiol 167:7–14

92. Humar B, Graziano F, Cascinu S et al (2002) Association of CDH1 haplotypes with susceptibility to sporadic diffuse gastric cancer. Oncogene 21:8192–8195
93. Nasri S, More H, Graziano F et al (2008) A novel diffuse gastric cancer susceptibility variant in E-cadherin (CDH1) intron 2: a case control study in an Italian population. BMC Cancer 8:138
94. Oliveira C, Bordin MC, Grehan N et al (2002) Screening E-cadherin in gastric cancer families reveals germline mutations only in hereditary diffuse gastric cancer kindred. Hum Mutat 19:510–517
95. Oliveira C, Senz J, Kaurah P et al (2009) Germline CDH1 deletions in hereditary diffuse gastric cancer families. Hum Mol Genet 18(9):1545–1555
96. Frebourg T, Oliveira C, Hochain P et al (2006) Cleft lip/palate and CDH1/E-cadherin mutations in families with hereditary diffuse gastric cancer. J Med Genet 43:138–142
97. Strachan T, Read A (2003) Human molecular genetics, 3rd edn. Garland Science, Oxford
98. Vleminckx K, Vakaet L Jr, Mareel M, Fiers W, van Roy F (1991) Genetic manipulation of E-cadherin expression by epithelial tumor cells reveals an invasion suppressor role. Cell 66:107–119
99. Perl AK, Wilgenbus P, Dahl U, Semb H, Christofori G (1998) A causal role for E-cadherin in the transition from adenoma to carcinoma. Nature 392:190–193
100. Bukholm IK, Nesland JM, Borresen-Dale AL (2000) Re-expression of E-cadherin, alpha-catenin and β-catenin, but not of gamma-catenin, in metastatic tissue from breast cancer patients [see comments]. J Pathol 190:15–19
101. Handschuh G, Candidus S, Luber B et al (1999) Tumour-associated E-cadherin mutations alter cellular morphology, decrease cellular adhesion and increase cellular motility. Oncogene 18:4301–4312
102. Becker KF, Atkinson MJ, Reich U et al (1994) E-cadherin gene mutations provide clues to diffuse type gastric carcinomas. Cancer Res 54:3845–3852
103. Machado JC, Oliveira C, Carvalho R et al (2001) E-cadherin gene (CDH1) promoter methylation as the second hit in sporadic diffuse gastric carcinoma. Oncogene 20:1525–1528
104. Moll R, Mitze M, Frixen UH, Birchmeier W (1993) Differential loss of E-cadherin expression in infiltrating ductal and lobular breast carcinomas. Am J Pathol 143:1731–1742
105. Vos CB, Cleton-Jansen AM, Berx G et al (1997) E-cadherin inactivation in lobular carcinoma in situ of the breast: an early event in tumorigenesis. Br J Cancer 76:1131–1133
106. Oliveira C, Sousa S, Pinheiro H et al (2009) Quantification of epigenetic and genetic second hits in CDH1 during hereditary diffuse gastric cancer syndrome progression. Gastroenterology 136(7):2137–2148
107. Yang J, Weinberg RA (2008) Epithelial-mesenchymal transition: at the crossroads of development and tumor metastasis. Dev Cell 14:818–829
108. Berx G, Cleton-Jansen AM, Nollet F et al (1995) E-cadherin is a tumour/invasion suppressor gene mutated in human lobular breast cancers. EMBO J 14:6107–6115
109. Christofori G, Semb H (1999) The role of the cell-adhesion molecule E-cadherin as a tumour-suppressor gene. Trends Biochem Sci 24:73–76
110. Oda T, Kanai Y, Oyama T et al (1994) E-cadherin gene mutations in human gastric carcinoma cell lines. Proc Natl Acad Sci U S A 91:1858–1862
111. Grady WM, Willis J, Guilford PJ et al (2000) Methylation of the CDH1 promoter as the second genetic hit in hereditary diffuse gastric cancer. Nat Genet 26:16–17
112. Barber M, Murrell A, Ito Y et al (2008) Mechanisms and sequelae of E-cadherin silencing in hereditary diffuse gastric cancer. J Pathol 216:295–306
113. Knudson AG Jr (1971) Mutation and cancer: statistical study of retinoblastoma. Proc Natl Acad Sci U S A 68:820–823
114. Orsulic S, Huber O, Aberle H, Arnold S, Kemler R (1999) E-cadherin binding prevents β-catenin nuclear localization and β-catenin/LEF-1-mediated transactivation. J Cell Sci 112(Pt 8):1237–1245

115. Aoki K, Taketo MM (2007) Adenomatous polyposis coli (APC): a multi-functional tumor suppressor gene. J Cell Sci 120:3327–3335
116. Novak A, Dedhar S (1999) Signaling through β-catenin and Lef/Tcf. Cell Mol Life Sci 56:523–537
117. He TC, Sparks AB, Rago C et al (1998) Identification of c-MYC as a target of the APC pathway. Science 281:1509–1512
118. Gottardi CJ, Gumbiner BM (2004) Distinct molecular forms of β-catenin are targeted to adhesive or transcriptional complexes. J Cell Biol 167:339–349
119. Barber M, Fitzgerald RC, Caldas C (2006) Familial gastric cancer – aetiology and pathogenesis. Best Pract Res Clin Gastroenterol 20:721–734
120. Geary J, Sasieni P, Houlston R et al (2007) Gene-related cancer spectrum in families with hereditary non-polyposis colorectal cancer (HNPCC). Fam Cancer 7(2):163–172
121. Douglas JA, Gruber SB, Meister KA et al (2005) History and molecular genetics of lynch syndrome in family G: a century later. JAMA 294:2195–2202
122. Cai SJ, Xu Y, Cai GX et al (2003) Clinical characteristics and diagnosis of patients with hereditary nonpolyposis colorectal cancer. World J Gastroenterol 9:284–287
123. Park YJ, Shin KH, Park JG (2000) Risk of gastric cancer in hereditary nonpolyposis colorectal cancer in Korea. Clin Cancer Res 6:2994–2998
124. Giardiello FM, Brensinger JD, Tersmette AC et al (2000) Very high risk of cancer in familial peutz-jeghers syndrome. Gastroenterology 119:1447–1453
125. Oliveira C, Ferreira P, Nabais S et al (2004) E-cadherin (CDH1) and p53 rather than SMAD4 and caspase-10 germline mutations contribute to genetic predisposition in Portuguese gastric cancer patients. Eur J Cancer 40:1897–1903
126. Keller G, Vogelsang H, Becker I et al (2004) Germline mutations of the E-cadherin(CDH1) and TP53 genes, rather than of RUNX3 and HPP1, contribute to genetic predisposition in German gastric cancer patients. J Med Genet 41:e89
127. Jagelman DG, DeCosse JJ, Bussey HJ (1988) Upper gastrointestinal cancer in familial adenomatous polyposis. Lancet 1:1149–1151
128. Shimoyama S, Aoki F, Kawahara M et al (2004) Early gastric cancer development in a familial adenomatous polyposis patient. Dig Dis Sci 49:260–265
129. Brose MS, Rebbeck TR, Calzone KA, Stopfer JE, Nathanson KL, Weber BL (2002) Cancer risk estimates for BRCA1 mutation carriers identified in a risk evaluation program. J Natl Cancer Inst 94:1365–1372
130. Cancer Risks in BRCA2 Mutation Carriers (1999) Cancer risks in BRCA2 mutation carriers the breast cancer linkage consortium. J Natl Cancer Inst 91:1310–1316
131. Risch HA, McLaughlin JR, Cole DE et al (2001) Prevalence and penetrance of germline BRCA1 and BRCA2 mutations in a population series of 649 women with ovarian cancer. Am J Hum Genet 68:700–710
132. Study Group of Millennium Genome Project for Cancer, Sakamoto H, Yoshimura K et al (2008) Genetic variation in PSCA is associated with susceptibility to diffuse-type gastric cancer. Nat Genet 40:730–740
133. JONES EG (1964) Familial gastric cancer. N Z Med J 63:287–296
134. Guilford PJ, Hopkins JB, Grady WM et al (1999) E-cadherin germline mutations define an inherited cancer syndrome dominated by diffuse gastric cancer. Hum Mutat 14: 249–255
135. Gayther SA, Gorringe KL, Ramus SJ et al (1998) Identification of germ-line E-cadherin mutations in gastric cancer families of European origin. Cancer Res 58:4086–4089
136. Richards FM, McKee SA, Rajpar MH et al (1999) Germline E-cadherin gene (CDH1) mutations predispose to familial gastric cancer and colorectal cancer. Hum Mol Genet 8:607–610
137. Shinmura K, Kohno T, Takahashi M et al (1999) Familial gastric cancer: clinicopathological characteristics, RER phenotype and germline p53 and E-cadherin mutations. Carcinogenesis 20:1127–1131

138. Yoon KA, Ku JL, Yang HK, Kim WH, Park SY, Park JG (1999) Germline mutations of E-cadherin gene in Korean familial gastric cancer patients. J Hum Genet 44:177–180

139. Ascano JJ, Frierson H Jr, Moskaluk CA et al (2001) Inactivation of the E-cadherin gene in sporadic diffuse-type gastric cancer. Mod Pathol 14:942–949

140. Dussaulx-Garin L, Blayau M, Pagenault M et al (2001) A new mutation of E-cadherin gene in familial gastric linitis plastica cancer with extra-digestive dissemination. Eur J Gastroenterol Hepatol 13:711–715

141. Yabuta T, Shinmura K, Tani M et al (2002) E-cadherin gene variants in gastric cancer families whose probands are diagnosed with diffuse gastric cancer. Int J Cancer 101:434–441

142. Humar B, Toro T, Graziano F et al (2002) Novel germline CDH1 mutations in hereditary diffuse gastric cancer families. Hum Mutat 19:518–525

143. Jonsson BA, Bergh A, Stattin P, Emmanuelsson M, Gronberg H (2002) Germline mutations in E-cadherin do not explain association of hereditary prostate cancer, gastric cancer and breast cancer. Int J Cancer 98:838–843

144. Sarrio D, Moreno-Bueno G, Hardisson D et al (2003) Epigenetic and genetic alterations of APC and CDH1 genes in lobular breast cancer: relationships with abnormal E-cadherin and catenin expression and microsatellite instability. Int J Cancer 106:208–215

145. Wang Y, Song JP, Ikeda M, Shinmura K, Yokota J, Sugimura H (2003) Ile-leu substitution (I415L) in germline E-cadherin gene (CDH1) in Japanese familial gastric cancer. Jpn J Clin Oncol 33:17–20

146. Jiang Y, Wan YL, Wang ZJ, Zhao B, Zhu J, Huang YT (2004) Germline E-cadherin gene mutation screening in familial gastric cancer kindreds. Zhonghua Wai Ke Za Zhi 42:914–917

147. Karam R, Carvalho J, Bruno I et al (2008) The NMD mRNA surveillance pathway downregulates aberrant E-cadherin transcripts in gastric cancer cells and in CDH1 mutation carriers. Oncogene 27:4255–4260

148. Lee JH, Han SU, Cho H et al (2000) A novel germ line juxtamembrane met mutation in human gastric cancer. Oncogene 19:4947–4953

149. More H, Humar B, Weber W et al (2007) Identification of seven novel germline mutations in the human E-cadherin (CDH1) gene. Hum Mutat 28:203

150. Kim IJ, Park JH, Kang HC et al (2003) A novel germline mutation in the MET extracellular domain in a Korean patient with the diffuse type of familial gastric cancer. J Med Genet 40:e97

151. Pinheiro H, Bordeira-Carrico R, Seixas S et al (2010) Allele-specific CDH1 downregulation and hereditary diffuse gastric cancer. Hum Mol Genet 19:943–952

152. Oliveira C, de Bruin J, Nabais S et al (2004) Intragenic deletion of CDH1 as the inactivating mechanism of the wild-type allele in an HDGC tumour. Oncogene 23:2236–2240

153. Vidal-Puig A, Moller DE (1994) Comparative sensitivity of alternative single-strand conformation polymorphism (SSCP) methods. BioTechniques 17:490–492, 494, 496

154. Mullins FM, Dietz L, Lay M et al (2007) Identification of an intronic single nucleotide polymorphism leading to allele dropout during validation of a CDH1 sequencing assay: implications for designing polymerase chain reaction-based assays. Genet Med 9:752–760

155. van Kouwen MC, Drenth JP, Oyen WJ et al (2004) [18F]fluoro-2-deoxy-D-glucose positron emission tomography detects gastric carcinoma in an early stage in an asymptomatic E-cadherin mutation carrier. Clin Cancer Res 10:6456–6459

156. Pacelli F, Papa V, Rosa F et al (2008) Four hundred consecutive total gastrectomies for gastric cancer: a single-institution experience. Arch Surg 143:769–775, discussion 775

157. Lynch HT, Kaurah P, Wirtzfeld D et al (2008) Hereditary diffuse gastric cancer: diagnosis, genetic counseling, and prophylactic total gastrectomy. Cancer 112:2655–2663

158. Kaurah P, Fitzgerald R, Dwerryhouse S et al (2010) Pregnancy after prophylactic total gastrectomy. Fam Cancer

159. Masciari S, Larsson N, Senz J et al (2007) Germline E-cadherin mutations in familial lobular breast cancer. J Med Genet 44(11):726–731

160. Schrader KA, Masciari S, Boyd N et al (2008) Hereditary diffuse gastric cancer: association with lobular breast cancer. Fam Cancer 7:73–82

161. Arpino G, Bardou VJ, Clark GM, Elledge RM (2004) Infiltrating lobular carcinoma of the breast: tumor characteristics and clinical outcome. Breast Cancer Res 6:R149–R156

162. Berx G, Van Roy F (2001) The E-cadherin/catenin complex: an important gatekeeper in breast cancer tumorigenesis and malignant progression. Breast Cancer Res 3:289–293

163. Berx G, Cleton-Jansen AM, Strumane K et al (1996) E-cadherin is inactivated in a majority of invasive human lobular breast cancers by truncation mutations throughout its extracellular domain. Oncogene 13:1919–1925

164. Droufakou S, Deshmane V, Roylance R, Hanby A, Tomlinson I, Hart IR (2001) Multiple ways of silencing E-cadherin gene expression in lobular carcinoma of the breast. Int J Cancer 92:404–408

165. Thull DL, Vogel VG (2004) Recognition and management of hereditary breast cancer syndromes. Oncologist 9:13–24

166. Rosman DS, Kaklamani V, Pasche B (2007) New insights into breast cancer genetics and impact on patient management. Curr Treat Options Oncol 8:61–73

167. Byrnes GB, Southey MC, Hopper JL (2008) Are the so-called low penetrance breast cancer genes, ATM, BRIP1, PALB2 and CHEK2, high risk for women with strong family histories? Breast Cancer Res 10:208

168. Smith RA, Saslow D, Sawyer KA et al (2003) American cancer society guidelines for breast cancer screening: update 2003. CA Cancer J Clin 53:141–169

169. Saslow D, Boetes C, Burke W et al (2007) American cancer society guidelines for breast screening with MRI as an adjunct to mammography. CA Cancer J Clin 57:75–89

170. Port ER, Park A, Borgen PI, Morris E, Montgomery LL (2007) Results of MRI screening for breast cancer in high-risk patients with LCIS and atypical hyperplasia. Ann Surg Oncol 14:1051–1057

171. Fisher B, Costantino J, Redmond C et al (1989) A randomized clinical trial evaluating tamoxifen in the treatment of patients with node-negative breast cancer who have estrogen-receptor-positive tumors. N Engl J Med 320:479–484

172. Land SR, Wickerham DL, Costantino JP et al (2006) Patient-reported symptoms and quality of life during treatment with tamoxifen or raloxifene for breast cancer prevention: the NSABP study of tamoxifen and raloxifene (STAR) P-2 trial. JAMA 295:2742–2751

173. Wolmark N, Dunn BK (2001) The role of tamoxifen in breast cancer prevention: issues sparked by the NSABP breast cancer prevention trial (P-1). Ann N Y Acad Sci 949:99–108

174. Rebbeck TR, Friebel T, Lynch HT et al (2004) Bilateral prophylactic mastectomy reduces breast cancer risk in BRCA1 and BRCA2 mutation carriers: the PROSE study group. J Clin Oncol 22:1055–1062

175. Barton MB, West CN, Liu IL et al (2005) Complications following bilateral prophylactic mastectomy. J Natl Cancer Inst Monogr(35):61–66

176. Lodder LN, Frets PG, Trijsburg RW et al (2002) One year follow-up of women opting for presymptomatic testing for BRCA1 and BRCA2: emotional impact of the test outcome and decisions on risk management (surveillance or prophylactic surgery). Breast Cancer Res Treat 73:97–112

177. Qiu LX, Li RT, Zhang JB et al (2009) The E-cadherin (CDH1) – 160 C/A polymorphism and prostate cancer risk: a meta-analysis. Eur J Hum Genet 17:244–249

Chapter 4
Genetics and Genomics of Neuroblastoma

Mario Capasso and Sharon J. Diskin

Abstract Neuroblastoma is a pediatric cancer of the developing sympathetic nervous system that most often affects young children. It remains an important pediatric problem because it accounts for approximately 15% of childhood cancer mortality. The disease is clinically heterogeneous, with the likelihood of cure varying greatly according to age at diagnosis, extent of disease, and tumor biology. This extreme clinical heterogeneity reflects the complexity of genetic and genomic events associated with development and progression of disease. Inherited genetic variants and mutations that initiate tumorigenesis have been identified in neuroblastoma and multiple somatically acquired genomic alterations have been described that are relevant to disease progression. This chapter focuses on recent genome-wide studies that have utilized high-density single nucleotide polymorphism (SNP) genotyping arrays to discover genetic factors predisposing to tumor initiation such as rare mutations at locus 2p23 (in *ALK* gene) for familial neuroblastoma, common SNPs at 6p22 (*FLJ22536* and *FLJ44180*) and 2q35 (*BARD1*), and a copy number polymorphism at 1q21.1 (*NBPF23*) for sporadic neuroblastoma. It also deals with well known and recently reported somatic changes in the tumor genome such as mutations, gain of alleles and activation of oncogenes, loss of alleles, or changes in tumor-cell ploidy leading to the diverse clinical behavior of neuroblastomas. Finally, this chapter reviews gene expression profiles of neuroblastoma associated with pathways of the signaling of neurotrophins and apoptotic factors that could have a role in neuroblastoma development and progression. Looking forward, a major challenge will be to understand how inherited genetic variation and acquired somatic alterations in the tumor genome interact to exact phenotypic differences in neuroblastoma, and cancer in general.

M. Capasso (✉)
CEINGE Advanced Biotechnologies, University of Naples "Federico II", Naples, Italy
e-mail: capasso@ceinge.unina.it

B. Pasche (ed.), *Cancer Genetics*, Cancer Treatment and Research 155,
DOI 10.1007/978-1-4419-6033-7_4, © Springer Science+Business Media, LLC 2010

1 Principal Concepts of Neuroblastoma

Neuroblastoma is a solid tumor that derives from primitive sympathetic neural precursors. About half of all neuroblastomas arise in the adrenal medulla, and the rest originate in paraspinal sympathetic ganglia in the chest or abdomen or in pelvic ganglia. Neuroblastomas account for 7–10% of all childhood cancers, and it is the most common cancer diagnosed during infancy [1]. The prevalence is about 1 case in 7,000 live births, and there are about 700 new cases per year in the United States [2]. This incidence is fairly uniform throughout the world, at least for industrialized nations. The median age at diagnosis for neuroblastoma patients is approximately 18 months; about 40% are diagnosed by 1 year of age, 75% by 4 years of age, and 98% by 10 years of age [3]. Age at diagnosis, clinical stage (based on the International Neuroblastoma Staging System [INSS]), and tumor histology are among the most important factors in predicting the outcome of the disease and accordingly modulate the treatment [4]. A hallmark of neuroblastoma is its clinical heterogeneity. In children over the age of 1 year, approximately 75% of cases present with disseminated metastases (stage 4); these tumors are aggressive, chemoresistant, and generally incurable. It is principally the dismal outlook for this group of patients that accounts for the disproportionate contribution of neuroblastoma to childhood cancer mortality (approximately 15% of cancer-related deaths). In contrast, infants with neuroblastoma tend to present with lower stage disease (stages 1, 2, and 4S), and the clinical behavior of these tumors differs greatly from the aggressive forms; they are generally chemosensitive and high cure rates are obtained. Moreover, a proportion of lower stage tumors show spontaneous regression, even those presenting with widespread dissemination in stage 4 disease. This extreme clinical heterogeneity reflects the complexity of genomic abnormalities acquired in tumor cells and has led some researchers to question whether neuroblastoma may consist of two distinctly different diseases.

This chapter reviews the genetics and genomics of this enigmatic tumor, emphasizing recently discovered germline mutations and common genetic variations that predispose to the development of this neoplasm and also reviewing somatic events associated with neuroblastoma pathogenesis and clinical phenotypes.

2 Genetics of Neuroblastoma Predisposition

2.1 Familial vs. Sporadic Neuroblastoma

Approximately 1% of neuroblastoma patients present with a family history of the disease [4]. Pedigrees from these rare families support an autosomal dominant mode of inheritance with incomplete penetrance [5]. Consistent with a cancer predisposition syndrome, familial neuroblastoma patients are often diagnosed at an earlier age and/or with multifocal primary tumors. Significant disease heterogeneity is observed, with both benign and malignant tumors often arising in the same family. Given that a common primary alteration is most likely shared among affected individuals in a family, it has been proposed that acquired secondary alterations ultimately define tumor phenotype [4, 6].

The vast majority of neuroblastomas arise sporadically, and the etiology is not well understood. The median age at diagnosis for sporadic neuroblastoma is 18 months, slightly higher than seen in familial neuroblastoma. Striking heterogeneity exists in terms of both tumor biology and clinical presentation. It is not uncommon for favorable tumors to spontaneously regress; however, the cure rate for children with more aggressive neuroblastoma is <30% despite intensive multimodal therapy. To date there have been no consistent reports of environmental factors contributing to neuroblastoma. Large constitutional chromosomal rearrangements have been observed in some neuroblastoma patients, including deletions overlapping putative tumor suppressor loci at chromosome bands 1p36 and 11q14–23 [7–9].

It has been thought for sometime that neuroblastoma predisposition is genetically heterogeneous and that initiation of tumorigenesis likely requires multiple alterations. The results of recent genome-wide efforts to identify familial and sporadic neuroblastoma predisposition genes strongly support this hypothesis and are the primary focus of this section.

2.2 Associated Conditions of Autonomic Nervous System: Shared Genetic Causes

Neuroblastoma patients sometimes present with associated conditions of the autonomic nervous system including congenital central hypoventilation syndrome, Hirschsprung disease, pheochromocytoma, and neurofibromatosis [10–13]. Comorbidities such as these suggest a common underlying genetic cause, and therefore genes involved in these disorders have been studied in neuroblastoma. Mutations in *PHOX2B* are commonly detected in congenital central hypoventilation syndrome [14, 15]. *PHOX2B* is a paired homeodomain transcription factor involved in the regulation of neurogenesis, and a small percentage of familial neuroblastoma cases (6.4%) have been shown to harbor loss-of-function mutations making *PHOX2B* the first bona fide neuroblastoma predisposition gene [16–18] (Table 4.1). Constitutional *PHOX2B* mutations have also been detected in a very small number of sporadic neuroblastoma patients; however, no somatically acquired alterations in primary tumors have been identified to date. Together, mutations in *PHOX2B* account for << 1% of neuroblastoma cases overall and are found almost exclusively in individuals with associated conditions of neural crest-derived tissues.

Table 4.1 Neuroblastoma genetic predisposition loci identified to date

Cytoband	Type	Identification	Gene(s)	Gene type	References
4p13	Rare mutation	Comorbidities	PHOX2B	Coding, tumor suppressor	[16–18]
2p23.1-.2	Rare mutation	Linkage	ALK	Coding, oncogene	[19, 47–49, 114]
6p22.3	Common SNP	GWAS	FLJ22536	Non-coding RNA	[27]
			FLJ44180	Coding, function unknown	[27]
2q35	Common SNP	GWAS	BARD1	Coding, cancer gene	[28]
1q21.1	Common CNV	GWAS	NBPF23	Coding, neurodevelopment	[30]

2.3 Familial Neuroblastoma Predisposition

The rarity and incomplete penetrance of familial neuroblastoma have made it difficult to study with traditional genetic approaches, until recently. Initial reports suggested that a hereditary predisposition locus mapped to the short arm of chromosome 16 (16p12–13); however, a specific gene mapping to this region has not be identified [3]. By performing a genome-wide scan for linkage at 6,000 single nucleotide polymorphisms (SNPs) using 20 neuroblastoma families, Mossé and colleagues recently identified a significant linkage signal on the short arm of chromosome 2 (2p23–p24) [19]. This locus included *MYCN*, a well-known oncogene in neuroblastoma; however, no sequence mutations were found in the coding or upstream regions of the gene. Ultimately, the anaplastic lymphoma kinase (*ALK*) gene which maps to 2p23 was identified as the major familial neuroblastoma predisposition gene [19] (Table 4.1). *ALK* is a receptor protein-tyrosine kinase which functions as an oncogene in many human cancers, most notably through translocations resulting in constitutive activation of the *ALK* kinase domain as seen in anaplastic large-cell lymphomas [20], inflammatory myofibroblastic tumors [21], squamous cell carcinomas [22], and non-small cell lung cancers [23, 24]. Resequencing of *ALK* coding exons in neuroblastoma probands revealed three distinct germline mutations within the tyrosine kinase domain, each with high probability for acting as oncogenic drivers [19, 25, 26] (Fig. 4.1). Notably, the few pedigrees of high confidence for heritability which did not have *ALK* mutations were found to harbor mutations in *PHOX2B* [19]. Contrary to *PHOX2B*, somatic alterations of *ALK* have been detected in primary neuroblastoma tumors (see Section 3.3), and a Phase I/II clinical trial of ALK inhibition therapy is ongoing in children with refractory disease.

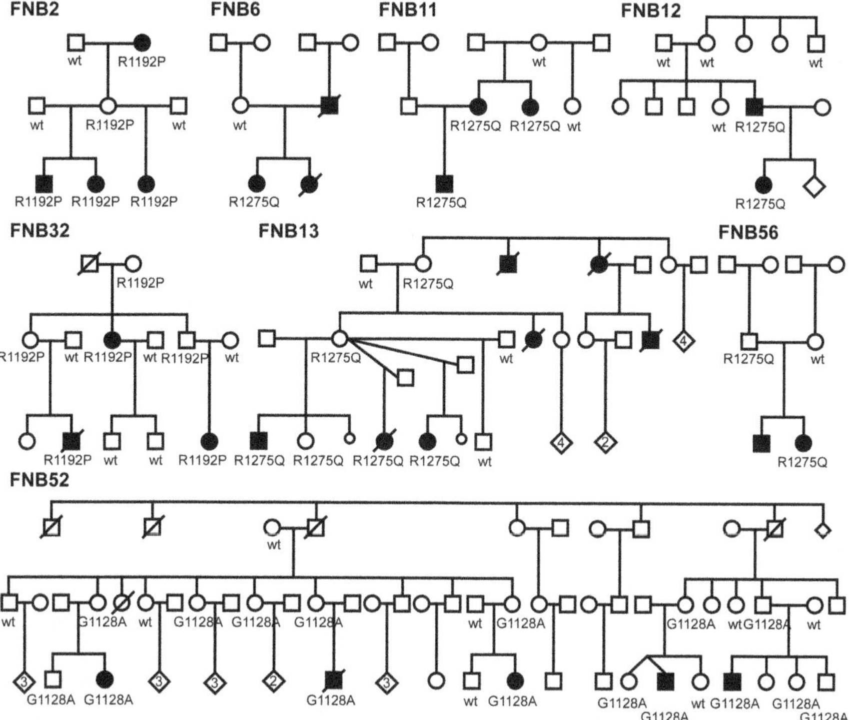

Fig. 4.1 Eight neuroblastoma pedigrees with ALK mutations. All family members with DNA available for genotyping are indicated either by wild type (WT) for *ALK* or by mutation in the *ALK* tyrosine kinase domain (R1192P, R1275Q, G1128A). Individuals affected by neuroblastoma are indicated by a *filled symbol*. The *numbers* inside the *small diamonds* indicate the number of other children, the *lines* through the *symbols* indicate that the person is deceased, and the smaller *circles* represent a miscarriage. Reprinted by permission from Macmillan Publishers Ltd: *Nature* [19], copyright 2008

2.4 Sporadic Neuroblastoma Predisposition

The genetic etiology of sporadic neuroblastoma is beginning to be unraveled. Our knowledge of complex diseases in general has increased substantially in recent years with the advent of affordable high-density SNP genotyping arrays and the accumulation of large banks of DNA from both affected and non-affected ("healthy") control populations. Genome-wide association studies (GWASs) comparing large populations of cases vs. controls have proven to be a powerful tool in identifying genetic risk factors in complex disease. The underlying hypothesis driving this approach is that multiple common genetic variations interact to predispose an individual to the development of disease. The success of this approach requires large numbers of both affected and non-affected ("healthy") individuals. The importance of centralized banking of blood and tumor specimens from neuroblastoma patients was recognized and put into place years ago given the rarity of the disease, and this helped position neuroblastoma to be the first childhood cancer to benefit from the GWAS approach.

2.4.1 Single Nucleotide Polymorphisms (SNPs)

The first report of a common genetic variant predisposing to a pediatric cancer came as the result of a GWAS of over 500,000 SNPs comparing blood DNA from nearly 2,000 Caucasian neuroblastoma patients to over 4,000 Caucasian cancer-free control subjects [27]. Maris and colleagues identified common SNPs at 6p22 within the predicted genes *FLJ22536* and *FLJ44180* associated with neuroblastoma (Table 4.1). Neuroblastoma patients homozygous for the risk alleles were more likely to have clinically aggressive neuroblastoma including metastatic disease at diagnosis, somatic amplification of the *MYCN* oncogene, and disease relapse. This work provided an important proof of principle for the GWAS approach to studying sporadic neuroblastoma susceptibility. It is not yet known how *FLJ22536* and/or *FLJ44180* influences the malignant transformation of developing neuroblasts.

The overrepresentation of 6p22 risk alleles in aggressive neuroblastoma was not completely unexpected and prompted a subsequent SNP-based GWAS focused specifically on the high-risk subset of neuroblastoma. A study of over 500 high-risk neuroblastoma cases and over 4,000 cancer-free control subjects confirmed the 6p22 signal described above and also revealed additional SNPs at 2q35 associated with aggressive neuroblastoma [28] (Fig. 4.2a). These SNPs were all located within *BARD1*, "*BRCA1*-associated RING domain 1." Evaluation of non-synonymous SNPs with the coding and upstream regions of *BARD1* in cases and controls identified additional SNPs significantly associated with neuroblastoma. *BARD1* has been previously implicated in several cancers due to its association with *BRCA1*, a well-known breast cancer susceptibility gene. *BARD1* heterodimerizes with *BRCA1* [29] and is thought to be necessary for the tumor suppressive function of *BRCA1*. Studies are ongoing to understand how sequence variations within *BARD1* influence neuroblastoma tumorigenesis. Together, the 6p22 and 2q35 associations suggest that genetic initiating events may predispose not only to neuroblastoma but to clinically relevant sub-phenotypes as well.

2.4.2 Copy Number Variations (CNVs)

In addition to SNP genotypes, copy number variations (CNVs) represent a significant source of genetic diversity that may influence disease susceptibility. The first definitive association of a germline CNV with human cancer came as the result of a CNV-based GWAS in neuroblastoma [30]. Researchers analyzed a total of 1,441 Caucasian neuroblastoma cases and 4,160 Caucasian controls and identified a common deletion polymorphism spanning less than 145 kb at 1q21.1 associated with neuroblastoma (Fig. 4.2b), no duplications reached genome-wide significance

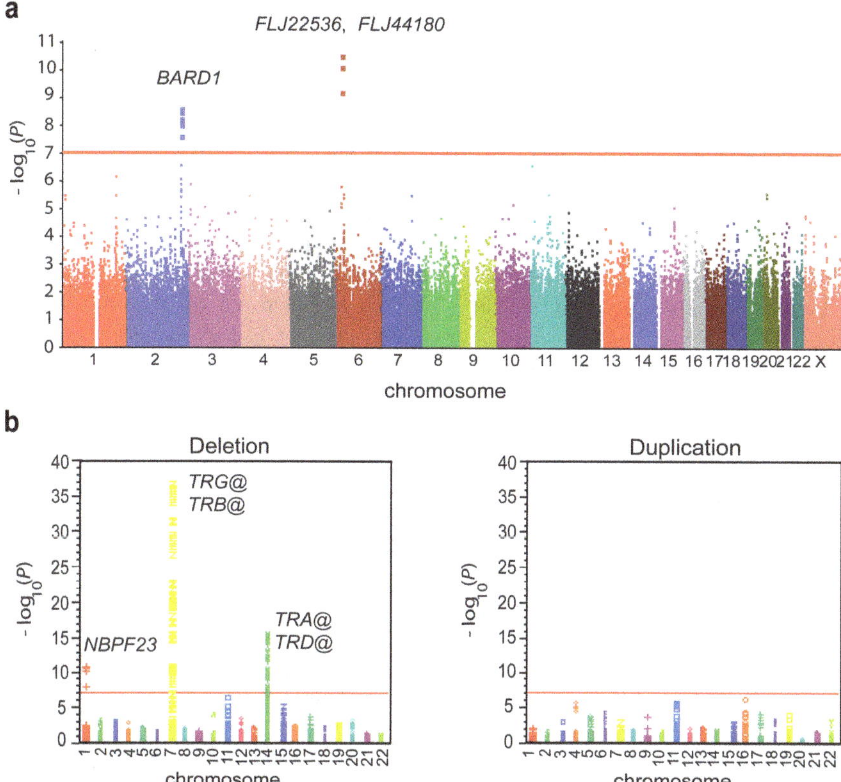

Fig. 4.2 Significant discovery findings from GWAS of SNPs and CNVs. (**a**) Summary of SNP-based GWAS results of high-risk neuroblastoma patients. Plotted are results from discovery set of 397 Caucasian high-risk cases and 2,043 Caucasian controls. *Y*-axis represents the level of significance for each SNP (log transformed *P* values) at the relative genomic position on each chromosome along the *x*-axis from short-arm terminus (*left*) to long-arm terminus (*right*). *Horizontal line* indicates threshold for genome-wide significance (*P* value $< 1 \times 10^{-7}$). Putative target genes are labeled at both the 6p22 and 2q35 loci. (**b**) Summary of CNV-based GWAS in neuroblastoma [30]. *Left*: deletions. *Right*: duplications. Plotted are results from discovery set of 846 Caucasian cases 803 Caucasian controls. *Y*-axis represents the level of significance for each SNP (log transformed *P* values) overlaid at each chromosome. *Horizontal line* indicates threshold for genome-wide significance (*P* value $< 1 \times 10^{-7}$). Putative target genes are labeled

(Fig. 4.2b) [30]. A novel member of the *NBPF* ("neuroblastoma breakpoint family") gene family mapping within the CNV was cloned and sequenced. Expression of this transcript, termed *NBPF23*, was found to be significantly correlated with the underlying CNV genotype in neuroblastoma tumors and cell lines, further supporting the biological relevance of the CNV association. Evaluation of *NBPF23* expression in a large panel of normal adult and fetal tissues revealed preferential expression in fetal brain and fetal sympathetic nervous tissues, consistent with *NBPF23* playing a role in early neuroblastoma tumorigenesis.

Notably, results of this CNV-based GWAS also revealed highly significant associations of deletion at all four T-cell receptor loci clustered on chromosomes 7 and 14 (Fig. 4.2b) [30]. These events were determined to be somatically acquired and likely represent an oligoclonal expansion of T-cell lymphocytes in the blood of neuroblastoma patients. T-cell receptor rearrangements were strongly associated with favorable features, and further investigation is warranted to determine if these events herald an immunologic response to neuroblastoma.

Together, these SNP and CNV associations support the hypothesis of multiple common genetic variants cooperating in the etiology of sporadic neuroblastoma. Remaining susceptibility loci will be identified as the result of ongoing GWAS efforts. Initial focus has been on Caucasian patients of European ancestry given that ~70% of neuroblastomas occur in this ethnic group; however, studies will expand to include other ethnicities as cases accrue and power to detect genome-wide significant associations is reached. In addition, data from GWAS efforts used to identify common genetic variants should also provide the means for investigating rare variants possibly conferring much greater risk.

2.5 *Model of Neuroblastoma Tumorigenesis*

Figure 4.3 illustrates a hypothetical model of neuroblastoma tumor initiation based on rare germline mutations and common genetic variations associated with the disease. The model is presented in terms of the number of co-occurring risk alleles (rare mutations and/or common genetic variations) in a child's germline DNA along with

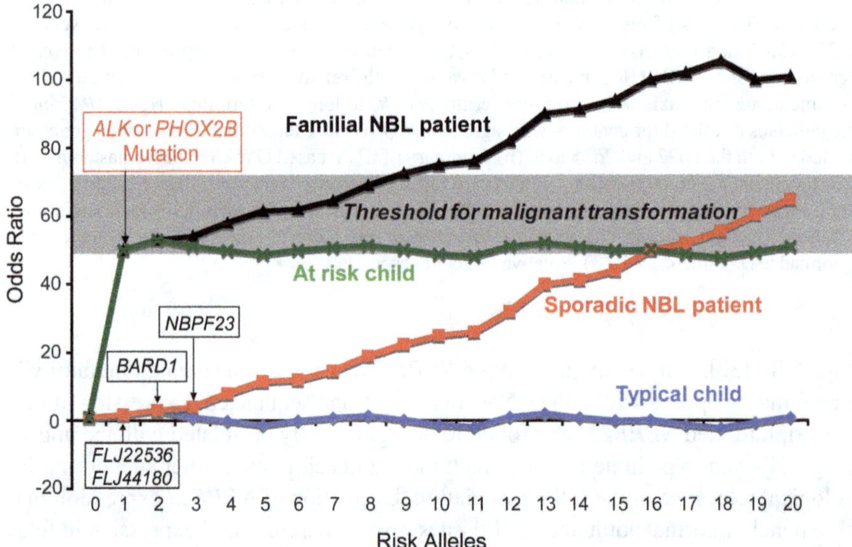

Fig. 4.3 Graphical model of the genetics of neuroblastoma tumorigenesis

the corresponding odds ratio assuming an additive effect. A threshold for malignant transformation is set at an odds ratio of approximately 50, as indicated in gray. A child with a germline *ALK* or *PHOX2B* mutation is at considerable risk for developing neuroblastoma. Based on the presence of additional risk alleles, this child may become a familial neuroblastoma patient (black); however, in the absence of additional risk alleles the child can remain at risk but not develop the disease (green). Conversely, a sporadic neuroblastoma patient lacking a germline mutation in *ALK* or *PHOX2B* likely requires the presence of 20 or more risk alleles in their germline DNA before reaching the threshold for malignant transformation (red). The typical child harbors only a small subset of neuroblastoma risk alleles in their germline DNA and thus is at no appreciable risk for developing the disease (blue).

3 Somatic Genetic Changes in Neuroblastoma

Somatic changes, such as mutations, gain of alleles, loss of alleles, or changes in tumor-cell ploidy, have been shown to be important in the development of neuroblastoma. Some of these abnormalities are powerful prognostic markers independent of clinical features. This fact helps in risk stratification of patients at presentation, with the most intensive treatments being reserved for high-risk cases, so that children with relatively benign tumors can be spared the deleterious effects of unnecessary chemotherapy.

3.1 Ploidy

Although many tumors have karyotypes in the diploid range, tumors from patients with lower stages of disease are often hyperdiploid or near-triploid [31, 32]. Studies by Look and colleagues have shown that determination of the ploidy status content of neuroblastomas from infants can be predictive of outcome [33, 34]. Unfortunately, ploidy loses its prognostic significance for patients who are older than 1–2 years of age [34]. This is probably because hyperdiploid and near-triploid tumors from infants generally have whole chromosome gains without structural rearrangements, whereas hyperdiploid/near-triploid tumors in older patients also have several structural rearrangements. Indeed, tumors showing no structural chromosomal changes but hyperdiploidy due to whole chromosome gains are more easily cured and may even spontaneously regress [35, 36].

3.2 *MYCN* Amplification

The genetic aberration most associated with poor outcome in neuroblastoma is genomic amplification of *MYCN* [37–39]. Schwab and colleagues in 1983 identified that *MYCN*, a gene located on the distal short arm of chromosome 2 (2p24), was amplified in a panel of neuroblastoma tumors and cell lines [40]. The process of amplification usually results in 50–400 copies of the gene per cell, with correspondingly high levels of protein expression [41]. Intermediate copy level numbers (i.e., 3–10 copies) may reflect either low-level amplification or aneuploidy. *MYCN* amplification occurs in roughly 20% of primary tumors and is strongly correlated with advanced stage disease and treatment failure [42, 43]. Its association with poor outcome in patients with otherwise favorable disease patterns such as localized tumors or INSS stage 4S disease underscores its biological importance [44–46]. In the United States, Europe, and Japan, assessing for the presence of *MYCN* amplification in neuroblastomas is currently and routinely included in the clinical practice because it is a powerful predictor of a poor prognosis.

3.3 *ALK* Amplification and Mutations

Somatically acquired gain and high-level amplification of the *ALK* locus have been identified as recurrent genomic abnormalities in neuroblastoma tumors and cell lines [19, 47, 48]. Resequencing of *ALK* coding exons in primary tumors and matched blood uncovered acquired somatic mutations consistent with those detected in the germline of familial neuroblastoma patients [19, 47, 49]; this work also led to the identification of constitutional *ALK* mutations in sporadic neuroblastoma patients [19, 47–49]. Mutated ALK proteins are overexpressed, hyperphosphorylated, and show constitutive kinase activity [19, 48, 49]. Targeted knockdown of *ALK* resulted in decreased cell proliferation in both *ALK*-mutated and *ALK*-amplified neuroblastoma cell lines, suggesting that *ALK* represents a promising candidate for targeted therapy in neuroblastoma [19, 47, 48]. Table 4.2 lists the known *ALK* mutations to date. Efforts are ongoing to fully define the spectrum and frequency of *ALK* sequence mutations and genomic amplifications in neuroblastoma and to understand the functional consequences of these alterations. Phase I/II clinical trial of ALK inhibition therapy is ongoing in children with refractory disease.

3.4 Amplification of Other Loci

In neuroblastoma cell lines or primary tumors amplification of at least six other regions that are non-syntenic with the *MYCN* locus at 2p24 has been shown. These include amplification of DNA from chromosomes 2p22 and 2p13, the *MDM2* gene on 12q13, and the *MYCL* gene at 1p32 [50–53]. Since these high-level amplifications usually appear concurrently with *MYCN* amplification, their prevalence, as well as biological and clinical significance, is unclear.

Table 4.2 *ALK* mutations identified in neuroblastoma patients

Mutation	Type	Location	References
R1275Q	Constitutional, somatic	TK domain	[19, 47–49, 114]
R1275L	n.d.	TK domain	[47]
F1174L	Somatic	TK domain	[19, 47–49, 114]
F1174I	Somatic	TK domain	[19, 114]
F1174C	Somatic	TK domain	[47, 49]
F1174V	Somatic	TK domain	[47, 49]
F1245C	Somatic	TK domain	[19, 48]
F1245L	Somatic	TK domain	[49, 114]
F1245V	Somatic	TK domain	[19, 48]
F1245I	n.d.	TK domain	[114]
D1091N	Somatic	N-terminal TK domain/ juxtamembrane	[19, 48]
A1234T	Somatic	TK domain	[48]
G1128A	Constitutional	TK domain	[19]
I1171N	Somatic	TK domain	[19]
I1250T	Somatic	TK domain	[19]
K1062M	n.d.	n.d.	[49]
M1166R	Somatic	TK domain	[19]
R1192P	Constitutional	TK domain	[19]
T1087I	Constitutional	upstream of TK domain	[49]
T1151M	Constitutional	TK domain	[48]
Y1278S	Somatic	TK domain	[47]

n.d.: not determined
TK: tyrosine kinase

3.5 Gain of 17q and Other Loci

In 1984 recurrent abnormalities of the long arm of chromosome 17 were first
identified by Gilbert and colleagues by using Giemsa-banded karyotypes derived
from primary neuroblastoma tumors and cell lines [54]. Allelotyping and CGH
studies have shown that this abnormality might occur in more than half of all neuroblastomas [55, 56]. Unbalanced gain of 17q often occurs through unbalanced
translocation with chromosome 1 or 11 [56]. The 17q breakpoints vary, but gain
of a region from 17q22-qter suggests that a dosage effect of one or more genes provides a selective advantage [57]. Candidate genes include *BIRC5* (survivin), *NME1*,
and *PPM1D*, which are overexpressed in this subset of tumors [58–60]. Gain of
17q is associated with more aggressive neuroblastomas, but its prognostic significance relative to other genetic and biological markers needs to be studied in a large
prospective trial and multivariate analysis. Common regional allelic gain at additional loci, including 1q, 2p, 11p, 11q, 12q, 18q, and other sites, has been identified
using comparative genomic hybridization (CGH) approaches [61–64].

3.6 Chromosome Deletion or Allelic Loss at 1p and 11q

There is a strong correlation between *MYCN* amplification and 1p loss of heterozygosity (LOH) that can be identified in 25–35% of neuroblastomas. Both *MYCN* amplification and deletion of chromosome 1p are strongly correlated with a poor outcome and with each other [51, 65–69]. However, the gene or genes within chromosome 1p involved in the pathogenesis of neuroblastoma have not been identified despite intensive investigation. Whether the loss of heterozygosity due to deletion of alleles from 1p is an independent indicator of prognosis remains controversial [35, 36, 70, 71]. A few studies suggest that allelic loss at 1p36 predicts an increased risk of relapse in patients with localized tumors [72–75].

Allelic loss of 11q detected by analysis of DNA polymorphisms and by CGH genomic aberration is rarely seen in tumors with *MYCN* amplification, yet remains highly associated with other high-risk features. Therefore, loss of 11q might prove to be useful predictor of outcome in clinically high-risk patients without *MYCN* amplification. In a study of almost 1,000 patients registered with Children's Oncology Group studies, unbalanced deletion of 11q (11q loss with either retention or gain of 11p material) was independently prognostic for outcome in a multivariate analysis [76]. Deletion of 11q was also directly associated with 14q deletion, but it was inversely correlated with 1p deletion and *MYCN* amplification [77].

There is evidence that LOH for the long arm of chromosome 14 occurs with increased frequency in neuroblastomas [78–80]. A deletion in 14q23-32 was found in 280 neuroblastomas but it was not associated with other biological or clinical features or outcomes [81]. Deletion or allelic loss has been shown at various other sites by genome-wide allelotyping or by CGH, but their biological or clinical significance is unclear.

4 Gene Expression Profiles of Neuroblastoma

Over the past 25 years, several gene expression studies have been performed using both neuroblastoma tumors and cell lines, and abnormal patterns have been identified. These findings suggest that pathways of the signaling of neurotrophins and apoptotic factors could have a role in neuroblastoma development and progression.

4.1 Neurotrophin Signaling Pathways

The factors that are responsible for regulating the malignant transformation of sympathetic neuroblasts to neuroblastoma cells are not well understood, but they probably involve one or more neurotrophin-receptor pathways that signal the cell to differentiate. Three tyrosine kinase receptors for a homologous family of neurotrophin factors have been cloned. The main ligands for the *TrkA*, *TrkB*, and *TrkC* (also known as *NTRK3*) receptors are nerve growth factor (*NGF*), brain-derived neurotrophic factor (*BDNF*), and neurotrophin-3 (*NT3*), respectively. Neurotrophin-4 (*NT4*, also known as *NT5*) also seems to function through *TrkB* [82, 83]. Binding of *TrkA* to a homodimer of *NGF* induces the activation of various signaling pathways linked to survival or to differentiation, whereas inhibition of *TrkA* activation can lead to programmed cell death, depending in part on the state of differentiation of the cell. So, the presence or absence of *NGF* can have a profound effect on cellular behavior.

A relationship between *TrkA* mRNA expression and patient survival in neuroblastomas and ganglioblastoma has been demonstrated. High levels of *TrkA* expression correlate with younger age, lower stage, and absence of *MYCN* amplification. In general, *TrkA* expression is associated with a favorable outcome, and the combination of *TrkA* expression and *MYCN* amplification provides a greater prognostic power. Other studies have demonstrated that full-length *TrkB* (there is also a truncated isoform lacking the tyrosine kinase) is expressed preferentially in advanced stage, *MYCN*-amplified neuroblastoma [84]. Many of these tumors also express *BDNF*, establishing an autocrine pathway promoting cell growth and survival [84, 85]. *TrkB* is expressed either in low amounts or as the truncated isoform in biologically favorable tumors. Lastly, *TrkC* is expressed in favorable neuroblastomas, essentially all of which also express *TrkA* [86–88].

Another transmembrane receptor called *p75* (*p75NTR*, also known as *TNFRSF16*) binds all the *NGF* family of neurotrophins with low affinity. This receptor is a member of the tumor necrosis factor receptor (*TNFR*) death-receptor. Theoretically, *p75* can lead to either cell death or differentiation in response to ligand, depending on whether or not *Trk* receptors are co-expressed [89, 90]. *p75* expression in neuroblastomas has generally been associated with a favorable outcome [91–93]. However, its biological and prognostic significance independent of *Trk* expression is unclear.

4.2 Apoptotic Signaling Pathways

Neuroblastoma has the highest rate of spontaneous regression observed in human cancers. Children with stage 4S neuroblastoma often have initial progression of multifocal disease followed by rapid tumor involution. Delayed implementation of normal apoptotic pathways has been proposed as an explanation for this phenomenon. Activation of programmed cell death can originate from various stimuli, such as the presence or absence of exogenous ligand or from DNA damage. However, members of the *TNFR* family (cell surface proteins), such as *p75* and *CD95*, might be involved in initiating apoptosis in neuronal cells and neuroblastomas [94–96]. The *BCL2* family of proteins responsible for relaying the apoptotic signal is highly expressed in most neuroblastomas, and the level of expression is inversely related to the proportion of cells undergoing apoptosis and the degree of cellular differentiation [97, 98]. The *BCL2* proteins might also be important in acquired resistance to chemotherapy [99, 100]. Ultimately, increased expression of caspases (proteins involved in the execution of the apoptotic signal) seems to be associated with favorable biological features and improved disease outcome [101]. So, neuroblastomas that are prone to undergoing apoptosis are more likely to spontaneously regress and/or respond well to chemotherapy.

4.3 Expression of Other Important Genes

Abnormal levels of genes resistant to several chemotherapeutic agents such as multidrug resistance gene 1 (*MDR*) and the gene for multidrug resistance-related protein (*MRP*) have been identified as predictors of therapy outcome for neuroblastoma [102–104].

Altered expression of the putative oncoprotein *NME1* (*NM23-H1*) that encodes the nucleoside diphosphate kinase A protein (*nm23A*) was noted in advanced (stages III and IV) primary neuroblastomas [105, 106], in a pattern opposite to that observed in other human malignancies. Chang and colleagues identified a ser120-to-gly (S120G) mutation in several high-grade neuroblastomas, but not in low-grade tumors or in control tissues [107].

Increased telomerase activity is detectable in most cancer cells and seems to be a prerequisite for malignant transformation [108]. Hiyama et al. were the first to show that telomerase expression was detectable in the vast majority of neuroblastomas (96%) [109]. In addition, very high levels of telomerase activity may correlate with adverse prognostic features and poorer survival probability [110–112]. Therefore, although elevated telomerase expression may simply be a marker of escape from cellular senescence, markedly increased levels may be associated with genomic instability and an increased likelihood of additional mutational events.

In 2006, Asgharzadeh and colleagues found that gene expression signatures of metastatic neuroblastomas that lack *MYCN* gene amplification identified two distinct groups of patients who were at low and high risk of disease progression [113]. Accurate identification of these subgroups with gene expression profiles may facilitate development, implementation, and analysis of clinical trials aimed at improving outcome.

4.4 Model of Neuroblastoma Subtypes

As initially proposed by Brodeur [6] there are at least two distinct types of neuroblastoma that are highly predictive of clinical behavior. Figure 4.4 presents a general model of neuroblastoma subtypes in relation to risk of death from disease. Newly diagnosed neuroblastomas can be divided into two broad subtypes characterized by the type of DNA copy number aberrations detected. The first type includes numerical aberrations where mitotic dysfunction leads to a hyperdiploid or near-triploid modal karyotype. These tumors harbor numerical chromosomal copy

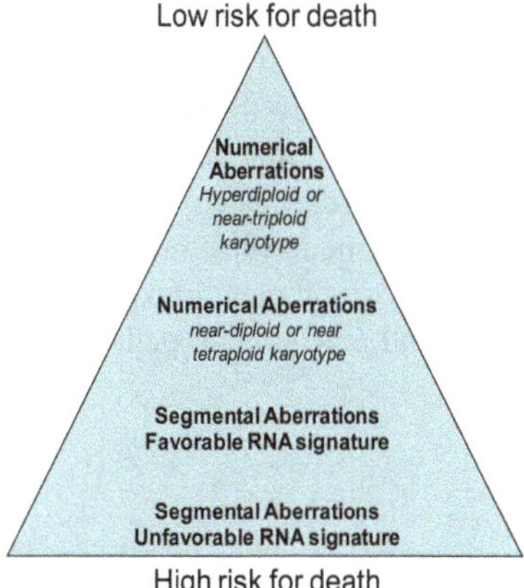

Fig. 4.4 Genomic model of neuroblastoma subtypes. In this general model, newly diagnosed neuroblastomas can be assessed for disease risk based on their underlying tumor DNA and RNA copy number profiles. It is proposed that a spectrum of risk exists ranging from the benign tumors harboring only numerical chromosomal aberrations to the highly malignant tumors with segmental chromosomal aberrations. This highly aggressive group is then subdivided based on "favorable" vs. "unfavorable" RNA signatures, where most *MYCN*-amplified tumors will have an unfavorable signature

number alterations and do not show specific structural genomic changes such as *MYCN* amplification and 1p LOH or 17q gain and generally express high levels of *TrkA*. Patients with type 1 tumors are usually cured with surgery alone and are generally less than 1 year of age with localized disease and a very good prognosis. The second broad type is characterized by segmental/structural chromosomal aberrations and these tumors generally have a near-diploid or tetraploid karyotype. No consistent abnormality has been identified, but 17q gain is most common, and high *TrkA* expression is rare. Within this type, two subsets can be distinguished based on tumor genomics. One subset is characterized by 11q deletion, 3p, 14q deletions or other changes, but they lack *MYCN* amplification and generally lack 1p LOH. Patients with these tumors are usually older with unfavorable outcome that is often fatal. The other aggressive group of tumors shows *MYCN* amplification, generally with 1p LOH. The age of these patients ranges from 1 to 5 years with advanced stage, rapidly progressive disease that is frequently fatal. Although these two groups are readily distinguished based on their profile of DNA copy number aberrations, it is proposed that risk of death is marked by RNA signatures. For this reason, the model presented in Fig. 4.4 divides the broad group of tumors with structural aberrations into those with favorable and unfavorable RNA signatures, where the tumors harboring segmental aberrations and an unfavorable RNA signature have the highest likelihood of resulting in a fatal outcome. Current research will address the specifics underlying this general model, with the goal of defining a set of tumor biologic features (DNA and RNA) for diagnostic use in neuroblastoma risk classification and ultimately treatment stratification.

5 Interaction of Germline Genetics and Tumor Genomics

Ongoing genome-wide studies are likely to identify additional germline risk alleles as well as somatically acquired genomic alterations in tumor cells. A challenge will be to understand the functional relevance of these findings within an integrated genetic and genomic landscape of neuroblastoma initiation and progression. It is anticipated that this will have a significant impact on unraveling the molecular mechanisms of tumorigenesis and new genetic pathways and targets of therapeutic agents in general.

References

1. Gurney JG et al (1997) Infant cancer in the U.S.: histology-specific incidence and trends, 1973 to 1992. J Pediatr Hematol Oncol 19:428–432
2. Brodeur GM, Maris JM (2006) Neuroblastoma. In: Pizzo PPD (ed) Principles and practice of pediatric oncology. J B Lippincott Company, Philadelphia, PA, pp 933–970
3. Brodeur GM, Maris JM (2002) Neuroblastoma. In: Pizzo P, Poplack D (eds) Principles and practices of pediatric oncology. J B Lippincott Company, Philadelphia, PA, pp 895–937
4. Maris JM, Hogarty MD, Bagatell R, Cohn SL (2007) Neuroblastoma. Lancet 369: 2106–2120
5. Knudson AG Jr, Strong LC (1972) Mutation and cancer: neuroblastoma and pheochromocytoma. Am J Hum Genet 24:514–532
6. Brodeur GM (2003) Neuroblastoma: biological insights into a clinical enigma. Nat Rev Cancer 3:203–216
7. Biegel JA et al (1993) Constitutional 1p36 deletion in a child with neuroblastoma. Am J Hum Genet 52:176–182
8. Satge D et al (2003) Abnormal constitutional karyotypes in patients with neuroblastoma: a report of four new cases and review of 47 others in the literature. Cancer Genet Cytogenet 147:89–98
9. Mosse Y et al (2003) Identification and high-resolution mapping of a constitutional 11q deletion in an infant with multifocal neuroblastoma. Lancet Oncol 4:769–771
10. Bower RJ, Adkins JC (1980) Ondine's curse and neurocristopathy. Clin Pediatr (Phila) 19:665–668
11. Maris JM, Chatten J, Meadows AT, Biegel JA, Brodeur GM (1997) Familial neuroblastoma: a three-generation pedigree and a further association with Hirschsprung disease. Med Pediatr Oncol 28:1–5
12. Knudson AG Jr, Meadows AT (1976) Developmental genetics of neuroblastoma. J Natl Cancer Inst 57:675–682
13. Knudson AG Jr, Amromin GD (1966) Neuroblastoma and ganglioneuroma in a child with multiple neurofibromatosis. Implications for the mutational origin of neuroblastoma. Cancer 19:1032–1037
14. Weese-Mayer DE et al (2003) Idiopathic congenital central hypoventilation syndrome: analysis of genes pertinent to early autonomic nervous system embryologic development and identification of mutations in PHOX2b. Am J Med Genet A 123A:267–278
15. Amiel J et al (2003) Polyalanine expansion and frameshift mutations of the paired-like homeobox gene PHOX2B in congenital central hypoventilation syndrome. Nat Genet 33:459–461
16. Mosse YP et al (2004) Germline PHOX2B mutation in hereditary neuroblastoma. Am J Hum Genet 75:727–730
17. Trochet D et al (2004) Germline mutations of the paired-like homeobox 2B (PHOX2B) gene in neuroblastoma. Am J Hum Genet 74:761–764

18. Raabe EH et al (2008) Prevalence and functional consequence of PHOX2B mutations in neuroblastoma. Oncogene 27:469–476
19. Mosse YP et al (2008) Identification of ALK as a major familial neuroblastoma predisposition gene. Nature 455(7215):930–935
20. Morris SW et al (1994) Fusion of a kinase gene, ALK, to a nucleolar protein gene, NPM, in non-Hodgkin's lymphoma. Science 263:1281–1284
21. Griffin CA et al (1999) Recurrent involvement of 2p23 in inflammatory myofibroblastic tumors. Cancer Res 59:2776–2780
22. Jazii FR et al (2006) Identification of squamous cell carcinoma associated proteins by proteomics and loss of beta tropomyosin expression in esophageal cancer. World J Gastroenterol 12:7104–7112
23. Soda M et al (2007) Identification of the transforming EML4-ALK fusion gene in non-small-cell lung cancer. Nature 448:561–566
24. Rikova K et al (2007) Global survey of phosphotyrosine signaling identifies oncogenic kinases in lung cancer. Cell 131:1190–1203
25. Torkamani A, Schork NJ (2007) Accurate prediction of deleterious protein kinase polymorphisms. Bioinformatics 23:2918–2925
26. Torkamani A, Schork NJ (2008) Prediction of cancer driver mutations in protein kinases. Cancer Res 68:1675–1682
27. Maris JM et al (2008) Chromosome 6p22 locus associated with clinically aggressive neuroblastoma. N Engl J Med 358:2585–2593
28. Capasso M et al (2009) Common variations in BARD1 influence susceptibility to high-risk neuroblastoma. Nat Genet 41:718–723
29. Wu LC et al (1996) Identification of a RING protein that can interact in vivo with the BRCA1 gene product. Nat Genet 14:430–440
30. Diskin SJ et al (2009) Copy number variation at 1q21.1 associated with neuroblastoma. Nature 18:987–991
31. Kaneko Y et al (1987) Different karyotypic patterns in early and advanced stage neuroblastomas. Cancer Res 47:311–318
32. Kaneko Y et al (1990) Current urinary mass screening for catecholamine metabolites at 6 months of age may be detecting only a small portion of high-risk neuroblastomas: a chromosome and N-myc amplification study. J Clin Oncol 8:2005–2013
33. Look AT, Hayes FA, Nitschke R, McWilliams NB, Green AA (1984) Cellular DNA content as a predictor of response to chemotherapy in infants with unresectable neuroblastoma. N Engl J Med 311:231–235
34. Look AT et al (1991) Clinical relevance of tumor cell ploidy and N-myc gene amplification in childhood neuroblastoma: a Pediatric Oncology Group study. J Clin Oncol 9:581–591
35. George RE et al (2005) Hyperdiploidy plus nonamplified MYCN confers a favorable prognosis in children 12 to 18 months old with disseminated neuroblastoma: a Pediatric Oncology Group study. J Clin Oncol 23:6466–6473
36. Janoueix-Lerosey I et al (2009) Overall genomic pattern is a predictor of outcome in neuroblastoma. J Clin Oncol 27:1026–1033
37. Schwab M, Tonini GP, Benard J (1993) Human neuroblastoma. Recent advances in clinical and genetic analysis. Harwood Academic Publishers, Chur, Switzerland, pp 101–111
38. Brodeur GM, Seeger RC (1986) Gene amplification in human neuroblastomas: basic mechanisms and clinical implications. Cancer Genet Cytogenet 19:101–111
39. Brodeur GM et al (1987) Consistent N-myc copy number in simultaneous or consecutive neuroblastoma samples from sixty individual patients. Cancer Res 47:4248–4253
40. Schwab M et al (1983) Amplified DNA with limited homology to myc cellular oncogene is shared by human neuroblastoma cell lines and a neuroblastoma tumour. Nature 305:245–248
41. Seeger RC et al (1988) Expression of N-myc by neuroblastomas with one or multiple copies of the oncogene. Prog Clin Biol Res 271:41–49

42. Seeger RC et al (1985) Association of multiple copies of the N-myc oncogene with rapid progression of neuroblastomas. N Engl J Med 313:1111–1116
43. Brodeur GM, Seeger RC, Schwab M, Varmus HE, Bishop JM (1984) Amplification of N-myc in untreated human neuroblastomas correlates with advanced disease stage. Science 224:1121–1124
44. Cohn SL et al (1995) Lack of correlation of N-myc gene amplification with prognosis in localized neuroblastoma: a Pediatric Oncology Group study. Cancer Res 55:721–726
45. Perez CA et al (2000) Biologic variables in the outcome of stages I and II neuroblastoma treated with surgery as primary therapy: a children's cancer group study. J Clin Oncol 18: 18–26
46. Katzenstein HM et al (1998) Prognostic significance of age, MYCN oncogene amplification, tumor cell ploidy, and histology in 110 infants with stage D(S) neuroblastoma: the pediatric oncology group experience – a pediatric oncology group study. J Clin Oncol 16:2007–2017
47. Janoueix-Lerosey I et al (2008) Somatic and germline activating mutations of the ALK kinase receptor in neuroblastoma. Nature 455:967–970
48. George RE et al (2008) Activating mutations in ALK provide a therapeutic target in neuroblastoma. Nature 455:975–978
49. Chen Y et al (2008) Oncogenic mutations of ALK kinase in neuroblastoma. Nature 455: 971–974
50. Brodeur GM, Maris JM, Yamashiro DJ, Hogarty MD, White PS (1997) Biology and genetics of human neuroblastomas. J Pediatr Hematol Oncol 19:93–101
51. Jinbo T, Iwamura Y, Kaneko M, Sawaguchi S (1989) Coamplification of the L-myc and N-myc oncogenes in a neuroblastoma cell line. Jpn J Cancer Res 80:299–301
52. Corvi R et al (1985) Non-syntenic amplification of MDM2 and MYCN in human neuroblastoma. Oncogene 10:1081–1086
53. Van Roy N et al (1995) Identification of two distinct chromosome 12-derived amplification units in neuroblastoma cell line NGP. Cancer Genet Cytogenet 82:151–154
54. Gilbert F et al (1984) Human neuroblastomas and abnormalities of chromosomes 1 and 17. Cancer Res 44:5444–5449
55. Caron H (1995) Allelic loss of chromosome 1 and additional chromosome 17 material are both unfavourable prognostic markers in neuroblastoma. Med Pediatr Oncol 24:215–221
56. Bown N et al (1999) Gain of chromosome arm 17q and adverse outcome in patients with neuroblastoma. N Engl J Med 340:1954–1961
57. Schleiermacher G et al (2004) Variety and complexity of chromosome 17 translocations in neuroblastoma. Genes Chromosomes Cancer 39:143–150
58. Islam A et al (2000) High expression of Survivin, mapped to 17q25, is significantly associated with poor prognostic factors and promotes cell survival in human neuroblastoma. Oncogene 19:617–623
59. Godfried MB et al (2002) The N-myc and c-myc downstream pathways include the chromosome 17q genes nm23-H1 and nm23-H2. Oncogene 21:2097–2101
60. Saito-Ohara F et al (2003) PPM1D is a potential target for 17q gain in neuroblastoma. Cancer Res 63:1876–1883
61. Brinkschmidt C et al (1997) Comparative genomic hybridization (CGH) analysis of neuroblastomas–an important methodological approach in paediatric tumour pathology. J Pathol 181:394–400
62. Lastowska M et al (1997) Comparative genomic hybridization study of primary neuroblastoma tumors. United Kingdom Children's Cancer Study Group. Genes Chromosomes Cancer 18:162–169
63. Vandesompele J et al (1998) Genetic heterogeneity of neuroblastoma studied by comparative genomic hybridization. Genes Chromosomes Cancer 23:141–152
64. Mosse YP et al (2007) Neuroblastomas have distinct genomic DNA profiles that predict clinical phenotype and regional gene expression. Genes Chromosomes Cancer 46:936–949
65. White PS et al (1995) A region of consistent deletion in neuroblastoma maps within human chromosome 1p36.2-36.3. Proc Natl Acad Sci U S A 92:5520–5524

66. White PS et al (2001) Detailed molecular analysis of 1p36 in neuroblastoma. Med Pediatr Oncol 36:37–41
67. White PS et al (2005) Definition and characterization of a region of 1p36.3 consistently deleted in neuroblastoma. Oncogene 24:2684–2694
68. Gehring M, Berthold F, Edler L, Schwab M, Amler LC (1995) The 1p deletion is not a reliable marker for the prognosis of patients with neuroblastoma. Cancer Res 55:5366–5369
69. Martinsson T, Sjoberg RM, Hedborg F, Kogner P (1995) Deletion of chromosome 1p loci and microsatellite instability in neuroblastomas analyzed with short-tandem repeat polymorphisms. Cancer Res 55:5681–5686
70. Schmidt ML et al (2005) Favorable prognosis for patients 12 to 18 months of age with stage 4 nonamplified MYCN neuroblastoma: a Children's Cancer Group Study. J Clin Oncol 23:6474–6480
71. Shimada H et al (1984) Histopathologic prognostic factors in neuroblastic tumors: definition of subtypes of ganglioneuroblastoma and an age-linked classification of neuroblastomas. J Natl Cancer Inst 73:405–416
72. Caron H et al (1996) Allelic loss of chromosome 1p as a predictor of unfavorable outcome in patients with neuroblastoma. N Engl J Med 334:225–230
73. Maris JM et al (2000) Loss of heterozygosity at 1p36 independently predicts for disease progression but not decreased overall survival probability in neuroblastoma patients: a Children's Cancer Group study. J Clin Oncol 18:1888–1899
74. Spitz R et al (2002) Fluorescence in situ hybridization analyses of chromosome band 1p36 in neuroblastoma detect two classes of alterations. Genes Chromosomes Cancer 34:299–305
75. George RE et al (2007) Genome-wide analysis of neuroblastomas using high-density single nucleotide polymorphism arrays. PLoS ONE 2:e255
76. Attiyeh EF et al (2005) Chromosome 1p and 11q deletions and outcome in neuroblastoma. N Engl J Med 353:2243–2253
77. Guo C et al (1999) Allelic deletion at 11q23 is common in MYCN single copy neuroblastomas. Oncogene 18:4948–4957
78. Srivatsan ES, Ying KL, Seeger RC (1993) Deletion of chromosome 11 and of 14q sequences in neuroblastoma. Genes Chromosomes Cancer 7:32–37
79. Carr J et al (2007) High-resolution analysis of allelic imbalance in neuroblastoma cell lines by single nucleotide polymorphism arrays. Cancer Genet Cytogenet 172:127–138
80. Suzuki T et al (1989) Frequent loss of heterozygosity on chromosome 14q in neuroblastoma. Cancer Res 49:1095–1098
81. Thompson PM et al (2001) Loss of heterozygosity for chromosome 14q in neuroblastoma. Med Pediatr Oncol 36:28–31
82. Yano H, Chao MV (2000) Neurotrophin receptor structure and interactions. Pharm Acta Helv 74:253–260
83. Patapoutian A, Reichardt LF (2001) Trk receptors: mediators of neurotrophin action. Curr Opin Neurobiol 11:272–280
84. Nakagawara A, Azar CG, Scavarda NJ, Brodeur GM (1994) Expression and function of TRK-B and BDNF in human neuroblastomas. Mol Cell Biol 14:759–767
85. Matsumoto K, Wada RK, Yamashiro JM, Kaplan DR, Thiele CJ (1995) Expression of brain-derived neurotrophic factor and p145TrkB affects survival, differentiation, and invasiveness of human neuroblastoma cells. Cancer Res 55:1798–1806
86. Svensson T et al (1997) Coexpression of mRNA for the full-length neurotrophin receptor trk-C and trk-A in favourable neuroblastoma. Eur J Cancer 33:2058–2063
87. Ryden M et al (1996) Expression of mRNA for the neurotrophin receptor trkC in neuroblastomas with favourable tumour stage and good prognosis. Br J Cancer 74:773–779
88. Yamashiro DJ, Nakagawara A, Ikegaki N, Liu XG, Brodeur GM (1996) Expression of TrkC in favorable human neuroblastomas. Oncogene 12:37–41
89. Casaccia-Bonnefil P, Gu C, Chao MV (1999) Neurotrophins in cell survival/death decisions. Adv Exp Med Biol 468:275–282

90. Hempstead BL (2002) The many faces of p75NTR. Curr Opin Neurobiol 12:260–267
91. Nakagawara A et al (1993) Association between high levels of expression of the TRK gene and favorable outcome in human neuroblastoma. N Engl J Med 328:847–854
92. Suzuki T, Bogenmann E, Shimada H, Stram D, Seeger RC (1993) Lack of high-affinity nerve growth factor receptors in aggressive neuroblastomas. J Natl Cancer Inst 85:377–384
93. Kogner P et al (1993) Coexpression of messenger RNA for TRK protooncogene and low affinity nerve growth factor receptor in neuroblastoma with favorable prognosis. Cancer Res 53:2044–2050
94. Brodeur GM, Castle VP (1999) Role of apoptosis in human neuroblastomas. In: Hickman JAD, Dive C (eds) Apoptosis and cancer chemotherapy. Humana, Totowa, NJ, pp 305–318
95. Bunone G, Mariotti A, Compagni A, Morandi E, Della Valle G (1997) Induction of apoptosis by p75 neurotrophin receptor in human neuroblastoma cells. Oncogene 14:1463–1470
96. Fulda S, Sieverts H, Friesen C, Herr I, Debatin KM (1997) The CD95 (APO-1/Fas) system mediates drug-induced apoptosis in neuroblastoma cells. Cancer Res 57:3823–3829
97. Castle VP et al (1993) Expression of the apoptosis-suppressing protein bcl-2, in neuroblastoma is associated with unfavorable histology and N-myc amplification. Am J Pathol 143:1543–1550
98. Oue T et al (1996) In situ detection of DNA fragmentation and expression of bcl-2 in human neuroblastoma: relation to apoptosis and spontaneous regression. J Pediatr Surg 31:251–257
99. Dole M et al (1994) Bcl-2 inhibits chemotherapy-induced apoptosis in neuroblastoma. Cancer Res 54:3253–3259
100. Dole MG et al (1995) Bcl-xL is expressed in neuroblastoma cells and modulates chemotherapy-induced apoptosis. Cancer Res 55:2576–2582
101. Nakagawara A et al (1997) High levels of expression and nuclear localization of interleukin-1 beta converting enzyme (ICE) and CPP32 in favorable human neuroblastomas. Cancer Res 57:4578–4584
102. Park JG, Kramer BS, Lai SL, Goldstein LJ, Gazdar AF (1990) Chemosensitivity patterns and expression of human multidrug resistance-associated MDR1 gene by human gastric and colorectal carcinoma cell lines. J Natl Cancer Inst 82:193–198
103. Chan HS et al (1991) P-glycoprotein expression as a predictor of the outcome of therapy for neuroblastoma. N Engl J Med 325:1608–1614
104. Norris MD et al (1996) Expression of the gene for multidrug-resistance-associated protein and outcome in patients with neuroblastoma. N Engl J Med 334:231–238
105. Hailat N et al (1991) High levels of p19/nm23 protein in neuroblastoma are associated with advanced stage disease and with N-myc gene amplification. J Clin Invest 88:341–345
106. Leone A et al (1993) Evidence for nm23 RNA overexpression, DNA amplification and mutation in aggressive childhood neuroblastomas. Oncogene 8:855–865
107. Chang CL et al (1994) Nm23-H1 mutation in neuroblastoma. Nature 370:335–336
108. Kim NW et al (1994) Specific association of human telomerase activity with immortal cells and cancer. Science 266:2011–2015
109. Hiyama E et al (1995) Correlating telomerase activity levels with human neuroblastoma outcomes. Nat Med 1:249–255
110. Hiyama E et al (1997) Telomerase activity in neuroblastoma: is it a prognostic indicator of clinical behaviour? Eur J Cancer 33:1932–1936
111. Reynolds CP et al (1997) Telomerase expression in primary neuroblastomas. Eur J Cancer 33:1929–1931
112. Brinkschmidt C et al (1998) Comparative genomic hybridization and telomerase activity analysis identify two biologically different groups of 4 s neuroblastomas. Br J Cancer 77:2223–2229
113. Asgharzadeh S et al (2006) Prognostic significance of gene expression profiles of metastatic neuroblastomas lacking MYCN gene amplification. J Natl Cancer Inst 98:1193–1203
114. Caren H et al (2008) High-resolution array copy number analyses for detection of deletion, gain, amplification and copy-neutral LOH in primary neuroblastoma tumors: four cases of homozygous deletions of the CDKN2A gene. BMC Genomics 9:353

Chapter 5
TGF-β Signaling Alterations and Colon Cancer

Naresh Bellam and Boris Pasche

Abstract Colorectal cancer is the second most common cause of cancer-related death in the United States. Twin studies suggest that 35% of all colorectal cancer cases are inherited. High-penetrance tumor susceptibility genes account for at most 3–6% of all colorectal cancer cases and the remainder of the unexplained risk is likely due to a combination of low to moderate penetrance genes. Recent genome-wide association studies have identified several SNPs near genes belonging to the transforming growth factor beta (TGF-β) superfamily such as *GREM1* and *SMAD7*. Together with the recent discovery that constitutively decreased *TGFBR1* expression is a potent modifier of colorectal cancer risk, these findings strongly suggest that germline variants of the TGF-β superfamily may account for a sizeable proportion of colorectal cancer cases. The TGF-β superfamily signaling pathways mediate many different biological processes during embryonic development, and in adult organisms they play a role in tissue homeostasis. TGF-β has a central role in inhibiting cell proliferation and also modulates processes such as cell invasion, immune regulation, and microenvironment modification. Mutations in the TGF-β type II receptor (*TGFBR2*) are estimated to occur in approximately 30% of colorectal carcinomas. Mutations in *SMAD4* and *BMPR1A* are found in patients with familial juvenile polyposis, an autosomal dominant condition associated with an increased risk of colorectal cancer. This chapter provides an overview of the genetic basis of colorectal cancer and discusses recent discoveries related to alterations in the TGF-β pathways and their role in the development of colorectal cancer.

Colorectal cancer is the fourth most common malignancy and the second most frequent cause of cancer-related death in the United States. In 2009, an estimated 146,970 cases of colorectal cancer were diagnosed and 49,960 people died from this

B. Pasche (✉)
Division of Hematology/Oncology, Department of Medicine, UAB Comprehensive Cancer Center,
The University of Alabama, Birmingham, AL 35294-3300, USA
e-mail: boris.pasche@ccc.uab.edu

B. Pasche (ed.), *Cancer Genetics*, Cancer Treatment and Research 155,
DOI 10.1007/978-1-4419-6033-7_5, © Springer Science+Business Media, LLC 2010

disease [1]. Institution of colonoscopy for at-risk individuals leads to earlier diagnosis of colon cancer which is amenable to curative surgery. Adjuvant therapy in patients with lymph node involvement has been demonstrated to have a benefit in overall survival [2]. Patients with widespread disease at diagnosis or with recurrent disease are treated with chemotherapy agents, although surgery with curative intent also has a role in the treatment of some patients with metastatic disease. The use of antibodies against vascular endothelial growth factor and epidermal growth factor results in a small but significant increase in the survival of patients with metastatic or recurrent colon cancer [3]. However, metastatic colorectal cancer is not a curable disease and therapy with current therapeutic agents is associated with significant morbidity.

The risk of developing colon cancer is approximately doubled in persons with a family history of colon cancer in a first-degree relative [4–6]. The risk increases with increasing number of first-degree relatives affected by colon cancer. Twin studies have suggested that genetic mutations contribute to the development of at least 35% of cases of CRC [7]. Hence, it is reasonable to estimate that at least one third of colon cancer cases are attributable to genetic factors.

1 Genetics of Colorectal Cancer

The most well-known familial genetic syndromes predisposing to the development of colorectal cancer are familial adenomatous polyposis and Lynch syndrome, formally named hereditary non-polyposis colon cancer. Familial adenomatous polyposis (FAP) is an autosomal dominant disorder that affects 1 in 13,000 births [8]. FAP is characterized by the formation of numerous polyps/adenomas throughout the large intestine in affected individuals, starting in their mid-twenties. The risk of these polyps/adenomas progressing to invasive carcinoma is 100%. Germline mutations in the adenomatous polyposis coli (*APC*) gene predispose individuals to develop numerous adenomatous polyps [9]. In addition, they have an increased risk of developing desmoid tumors, thyroid cancer, gastric adenocarcinoma, duodenal adenocarcinoma, and/or ampullary carcinoma. A missense mutation in the *APC* gene known as I1307K (isoleucine changes to lysine) is associated with colon polyps and an increased risk (up to 1.5–2 times) of developing colon carcinoma. The mutation leads to a hypermutable region, thereby indirectly predisposing to cancer. Importantly, this allele is found in 6% of Ashkenazi Jews but at a very low level in the general population [10, 11].

Lynch syndrome, formerly named hereditary non-polyposis colon cancer (HNPCC), is an autosomal dominant condition characterized by early onset of colon cancer. The average age at diagnosis is 45 years, the tumors tend to develop in the proximal colon and show evidence of microsatellite instability (MSI) [9]. Germline mutations in the DNA mismatch repair (MMR) enzymes predispose individuals to this syndrome. Deficiencies in these enzymes lead to numerous errors in DNA replication, especially in tandem repeat sequences, and cause lengthening of microsatellite sequences. Mutations in critical genes like *BAX*, *TGFBR2*, and *E2F4* can then initiate or promote carcinogenesis [12, 13]. Patients have an 80% lifetime risk of developing colon cancer and an increased predilection to develop extra-intestinal tumors in the endometrium, ovary, stomach, small bowel, hepatobiliary tract, pancreas, upper uroepithelial tract, and brain [14].

Deficiency in the base excision repair gene *MUTYH* also predisposes to colon cancer [13]. The *MUTYH* syndrome is inherited as a recessive trait and biallelic mutation carriers have almost a 100% risk of developing cancer. Variants in the *MUTYH* gene were identified in a family affected with multiple colorectal adenomas and carcinomas. Tumors from these individuals showed a predominance of somatic mutations in the *APC* gene. The majority of these *APC* mutations were G:C→A transversions, which suggests a defect in the base excision repair machinery [15]. It has been proposed that monoallelic mutations in the *MUTYH* gene also confer an elevated risk of colorectal cancer, although this is controversial [16–23]. A large population-based series of 9,628 patients with colorectal cancer and 5,064 controls were genotyped for *MUTYH* variants associated with colorectal cancer [24]. Biallelic mutation status was associated with a 28-fold increase in colorectal cancer risk (95% CI, 17.66–44.06). Monoallelic mutation was not associated with an increased colorectal cancer risk. Cancers associated with *MUTYH* mutations are thought to progress through a MSI-independent pathway [25]. It has not yet been fully determined as to why the *MUTYH* mutations predispose to the development of colorectal cancer [26].

The above-described mutations have a high penetrance with respect to colorectal cancer risk but, collectively, these various syndromes account for at most 3–6% of all colorectal cancers [27]. The remaining fraction of familiar cancers and a majority of sporadic cancers are likely to be due to low-penetrance mutations, i.e., mutations that have low frequency of association with a specific phenotype [9]. Genome-wide association studies have identified new genomic loci associated with colorectal cancer risk. A locus at 8q24 has been associated with a combined odds ratio of 1.17 (95% CI, 1.12–1.23; $p = 3.16 \times 10^{-11}$) [28, 29]. The association was confirmed in both sporadic and familial colorectal cancer. Single nucleotide polymorphisms (SNPs) near *GREM1*, *SCG5* [30], and *SMAD7* [31] genes have also been found to be strongly associated with colorectal cancer risk. Other genomic loci associated with an increased risk of developing colorectal cancer have been identified at 18q21, 8q23.3, 10p14, 11q23, 14q22.2, 16q22.1, 19q13.1, and 20p12.3 [29, 32, 33].

Gene polymorphisms in specific signaling pathways have also been shown to modify the risk of colorectal cancer. Epidemiological studies have shown an association between colorectal cancer, obesity, and insulin resistance. Elevated circulating levels of C-peptide and insulin-like growth factor binding protein I (IGFBP1) are directly associated with colorectal cancer risk [34–43]. Adiponectin, an endogenous insulin sensitizer, is a protein secreted by the adipose tissue. Adiponectin levels are decreased in patients with obesity and insulin resistance. A prospective clinical trial has demonstrated that men in the highest quintile of adiponectin levels have a decreased colorectal cancer risk when compared to men in the lowest quintile (relative risk, 0.42; 95% CI, 0.23–0.78) [39]. The hypothesis that genetic polymorphisms in the adiponectin gene *(ADIPOQ)* and its type I receptor *(ADIPOR1)* may affect the risk of colorectal cancer was examined by testing for differences in single nucleotide polymorphisms of the respective genes. Genotyping of haplotype tagging SNPs of the *ADIPOQ* and *ADIPOR* genes in two case–control studies with a combined population of 640 patients and 857 controls showed that one *ADIPOQ* SNP (rs266729), tagging the 5′ end of the gene, is consistently associated with a decreased risk of colorectal cancer after adjustment for age, sex, race, and SNPs within the same gene (adjusted odds ratio, 0.73; 95% CI, 0.53–0.99) [44]. An attempt at replicating these findings was recently conducted by Carvajal-Carmona et al. in two separate cohorts from the UK [45]. The association of the *ADIPOQ* genomic region with colorectal cancer was studied using the Illumina Hap 300/370/550 arrays that genotype 82 markers covering 250 kb around the *ADIPOQ* gene, none of which includes the rs266729 SNP. This study did not find an association between any of these SNPs with colorectal cancer risk. However, the r^2 value of the Illumina array SNP in strongest linkage disequilibrium with rs266729 was only 0.74. Furthermore, this SNP was located more than 7.7 kb upstream of rs266729. Thus, it is questionable that the Illumina array genotyping results truly excluded an association between rs266729 and colorectal cancer.

Adenomatous polyps have long been considered neoplastic lesions leading to the development of colorectal carcinoma. Another type of polyps, the hyperplastic (or serrated) polyps, have been regarded primarily as non-neoplastic polyps with no malignant potential of their own. However, several studies suggest that at least some serrated polyps may have malignant potential [46–48]. These serrated polyps named sessile serrated adenomas (SSA) [49] and dysplastic forms named serrated adenomas or SA [50] increase the likelihood of malignant transformation.

Genetic alterations observed in the sessile serrated adenomas and the serrated adenomas are different from those seen in the adenoma–carcinoma sequence [51–53]. For example, alterations in *TP53* and *APC* and loss of heterozygosity are rare, whereas alterations in microsatellite sequences and hypermethylation of CpG islands are common. Sessile serrated adenomas are associated with mutations in *BRAF* and show high levels of CpG island methylation. These adenomas only rarely have *KRAS* mutations [54–57]. Traditional serrated adenomas also show high levels of CpG island methylation but contain *KRAS* mutations more often than *BRAF* mutations [20, 57, 58]. Importantly, *KRAS* mutations and *BRAF* mutations have been found to be mutually exclusive [20, 59, 60].

Germline mutations in the TGF-β pathway are commonly found in patients diagnosed with familial juvenile polyposis (FJP), an autosomal dominant condition affecting 1 in 100,000 births [12]. It is characterized by the presence of 10 or more juvenile polyps in the gastrointestinal tract. Patients have an increased risk of colon cancer, even though estimates of cancer incidence have varied in different studies [61]. Mutations in the *SMAD4* and *BMPR1A* genes have been identified in FJP patients and account for about half of FJP cases [62–64]. Additional mutations have been described in the endoglin gene *(ENG)*, a co-receptor for TGF-β family receptors, but a causative role in FJP has not been conclusively proven [65]. In addition to the germline alterations that confer an increased risk of colorectal cancer, alterations in the TGF-β pathway have been documented in a high percentage of sporadic colon carcinomas. These mutations have been documented in both carcinomas with microsatellite instability (MSI) and carcinomas with chromosomal instability [66]. In this chapter, we will discuss the TGF-β signaling pathway alterations reported in colorectal cancer as well as our current understanding of the contribution of these alterations to colorectal carcinogenesis. A better understanding of this central pathway in colorectal carcinogenesis will be required to develop screening strategies and targeted therapies.

2 Overview of the TGF-β Pathway

TGF-β is a multifunctional cytokine with diverse effects on virtually all cell types and with key roles during embryonic development and tissue homeostasis [67]. Members of the TGF-β superfamily ligands, such as TGF-β, activin, and BMP, transduce their signals through heterotetrameric complexes comprising two types of serine–threonine kinase receptors, the type 1 and type 2. Upon ligand binding, the type 2 receptor phosphorylates and activates the type 1 receptor, which in turn initiates downstream signaling by phosphorylating the receptor-regulated SMADs (R-SMADs). Specific ligands signal through a specific combination of type 2, type 1, and R-Smads [68]. TGF-β binds to the TGF-β type 2 receptor (TGFBR2) and the TGF-β type 1 receptor (TGFBR1, formerly named TβRI or Alk5 for activin receptor-like kinase 5), although in endothelial cells it can also bind a complex comprising TGFBR2, ACVRL1, and TGFBR1 [69]. The type I receptor dictates the specificity for the R-SMADs: TGFBR1, ACVR1B, and ACVR1C phosphorylate SMAD2 and SMAD3, whereas ACVRL1, ACVR1, BMPR1A, and BMPR1B phosphorylate SMAD1, SMAD5, and SMAD8. Once phosphorylated, these R-SMADs transduce the signal to the nucleus in cooperation with the common mediator SMAD, SMAD4, to transcriptionally activate or repress different targets genes [68]. The SMAD4–R-SMAD complex has DNA binding capacity but association with additional DNA binding cofactors dictates which set of genes are transcriptionally regulated by this complex. The TGF-β superfamily pathways are also negatively regulated. The inhibitory SMADs, SMAD6 and SMAD7, bind the active receptor complexes and also recruit E3 ubiquitin ligase SMURF1/2 to the receptor complexes to degrade them [70, 71]. SMAD7 has also been shown to participate in a complex that dephosphorylates the active TGF-β receptor [72].

The TGF-β superfamily signaling pathways are involved in many different biological processes during embryonic development, and in adult organisms they play a role in tissue homeostasis [73]. TGF-β has a role in inhibiting cell proliferation but also modulates processes such as cell invasion, immune regulation, and microenvironment modification. It is generally accepted that excessive production and/or activation of TGF-β by tumor cells can foster cancer progression by mechanisms that include an increase in tumor neoangiogenesis and extracellular matrix production, upregulation of proteases surrounding tumors, and inhibition of

immune surveillance in the cancer host [74]. They are also strongly implicated in cancer, since alterations of some specific and some common components of these different pathways have been identified in the majority of human
tumors.

Two distinct types of genetic alterations have been identified: gain-of-functions
in oncogenes that usually result in growth factor-independent cell proliferation
and recessive loss-of-function mutations in tumor suppressors that allow evasion
of growth inhibitory signals. The well-characterized growth inhibitory response of
TGF-β [67], combined with the fact that up to 74% of colon cancer cell lines and
85% of lung cancer cell lines have become resistant to TGF-β antiproliferative effect
[75, 76], led several groups to search for evidence of inactivation of components of
the TGF-β pathway in human cancer.

Signaling alterations in the stromal compartment of tumors also have a pro-
tumorigenic effect. It has been found that TGF-β secretion is abundant in many
human cancers and the TGF-β-rich microenvironment is associated with poor prognosis, tumor vascularization, and metastasis [77]. TGF-β plays an important role
in the process of epithelial mesenchymal transition, myofibroblast generation, production of autocrine mitogens, and evasion of tumor immunity [74]. The role of
TGF-β signaling in the stromal compartment is of importance in processes important for carcinogenesis. Conditional knockout of *Tgfbr2* (type 2 receptor) in mouse
fibroblasts [78] led to hyperplasia in the adjacent epithelial tissue with subsequent progression to prostate intraepithelial neoplasia and gastric squamous cancer,
respectively. These *Tgfbr2*-defective fibroblasts had increased levels of hepatocyte
growth factor associated with increased activation of the hepatocyte growth factor
receptor, Met in adjacent tissues. Disruption of the TGF-β pathway in fibroblasts
leads to increased fibroblast proliferation and has been shown to promote mammary
tumor metastasis in fibroblast-epithelial cell cotransplantation studies in mice [79].

Other crucial functions of TGF-β related to cancer development and progression are its ability to suppress immune and inflammatory responses. TGF-β acts
as a central inhibitor of the multiple components of the native and the adaptive
immune system. It also stimulates the generation of T-regulatory cells, which inhibit
effector T-cell functions and IL-17 producing Th17 cells, which regulate NK cells
and macrophages [74]. These actions result in a context-dependent effect. *Smad3*
knockout mice develop colon cancers only after they are removed from a germ-free
environment or infected with *Helicobacter* spp. [80]. Conditional deletion of *Smad4*
in T cells has been associated with the development of colon carcinomas, and these
lesions are heavily infiltrated with plasma cells [81]. The loss of *Smad4* expression results in skewed maturation toward a *Th2* phenotype, with increased levels
of cytokines including IL-4,-5,-6, and -13 in vivo and in vitro. Knockout mice pro-
duced through expression of Cre under control of the designed promoter went on
to spontaneously develop carcinoma in the gastrointestinal tract. In addition, these
mice also exhibit a high rate of oral squamous cell carcinoma [81]. The chronic
inflammation induced in these experimental systems by the loss of TGF-β favors
tumorigenesis. On the other hand overexpression of TGF-β in certain tumors can
lead to evasion from the immune system and have a pro-tumorigenic role. TGF-β

also plays a role in epithelial mesenchymal transition (EMT) in human cancer [82]. EMT is a well-coordinated process during embryonic development and a pathological feature in neoplasia and fibrosis [83]. Cells undergoing EMT lose expression of E-cadherin and other components of epithelial junctions, produce a mesenchymal cell cytoskeleton, and acquire motility and invasive properties. It was first reported in mouse heart formation and palate fusion, in some mammary cell lines, and in mouse models of skin carcinogenesis that TGF-β is a potent inducer of EMT [83, 84]. TGF-β-induced EMT is observed in transformed epithelial progenitor cells with tumor propagating ability [85]. EMT-like processes contribute to tumor invasion and dissemination owing to the cell junction free, motile phenotype they confer. Carcinoma cells with mesenchymal traits have been observed in the invasion front of carcinomas and may reflect a series of interconnected features: that carcinomas are propagated by transformed progenitor cells, that progenitor cells are competent to undergo EMT, that EMT is triggered at the invasion front, which ultimately augments the disseminative capacity of these cells [74, 85]. TGF-β promotes EMT by a combination of SMAD-dependent transcriptional events and SMAD-independent effects on cell junction complexes. SMAD-mediated expression of HMGA2 (high mobility group A2) induces expression of SNAIL, SLUG, and TWIST [86, 87]. Independent of SMAD activity, TGFBR2-mediated phosphorylation of PAR6 promotes the dissolution of cell junction complexes [88]. In mouse tumors and cell lines, TGF-β-induced EMT is Smad-dependent and enhanced by Ras signaling [84]. TGF-β also enhances cell motility by cooperating with ERBB2 signals, as observed in breast cancer cells overexpressing ERBB2 [89].

3 TGF-β Signaling Alterations in Colorectal Cancer

3.1 Alterations in TGFBR2

Mutations in *TGFBR2* are the most common mechanism of loss of TGF-β signaling in colorectal cancer. It is estimated that approximately 30% of colorectal cancers harbor mutations in *TGFBR2* [76, 90]. The *TGFRB2* gene has a microsatellite sequence comprising an A(10) tract in exon 3 and GT(3) tracts in exons 5 and 7 called BAT-RII. These regions, especially the A(10) region, are prone to develop frameshift mutations in the presence of mutations in the DNA mismatch repair machinery. Almost 80–90% of colorectal tumors with microsatellite instability have mutations in *TGFBR2* [91, 92]. Other poly(A) tracts of similar length are mutated in these tumors, but not as frequently as *TGFBR2*. It is commonly speculated that colorectal cancers acquire partial TGF-β resistance largely because of *TGFBR2* genetic alterations. Interestingly, some colorectal cancer cell lines, which harbor homozygous mutations of *TGFBR2*, are growth-inhibited by TGF-β, which suggests that under certain circumstance, the cells can bypass *TGFBR2* to retain TGF-β-mediated growth inhibition [93]. Whether *TGFBR2* mutations have a causative role in colorectal carcinogenesis or whether they arise because of the hypermutable phenotype observed in cells with defective mismatch repair machinery is still a topic of debate. Fifteen percents of colorectal cancer cell lines without any evidence of microsatellite instability also harbor mutations in *TGFBR2* [76]. The effect of *Tgfbr2* loss in the intestinal epithelium in cancer formation was studied in a *Tgfbr2* conditional knockout mouse model. Azoxymethane (AOM) was used to induce colon cancer. Adenoma and carcinoma formation were significantly increased and increased neoplastic proliferation was noted in the mice devoid of *Tgfbr2* in the colonic epithelium ((4xat-132) Cre-Tgfbr2(flx/flx)) when compared with *Tgfbr2*(flx/flx) mice, which have intact *Tgfbr2* in the colon epithelium. The increased proliferation suggested that loss of TGF-β-mediated growth inhibition contributes to carcinogenesis. The increased proliferation noted could be due to the failure to inactivate Cdk4 expression as Cdk4 expression is upregulated in MSI+ cancers [94]. In addition, reconstitution of *TGFBR2* expression in a colon cancer line with known microsatellite instability was associated with decreased proliferation and decreased Cdk4 expression and kinase activity [94].

Studies evaluating the effect of *TGFBR2* mutations on the prognosis of patients with colorectal cancer have yielded conflicting results. The 5-year survival rate of patients with resected stage III colon cancer treated with adjuvant therapy was significantly higher in patients whose tumors exhibited microsatellite instability and *TGFBR2* mutations (74%) when compared to patients whose tumors had microsatellite instability without evidence of *TGFBR2* mutations (46%) [95]. On the other hand, a population-based study evaluating the impact of *TGFBR2* mutations on prognosis in MSI-positive tumors failed to reveal any significant difference in the age- and stage-adjusted risk of death associated with *TGFBR2* mutations in unstable tumors (138 out of 174) when compared to unstable tumors without such mutations [96]. However, another larger retrospective study suggested that *TGFBR2* mutations are not associated with prognosis in patients with high-microsatellite instability (MSI-H) tumors [97].

4 *TGFBR1* Mutations and Polymorphisms in Colorectal Cancer

Mutations in *TGFBR1* have been identified in human colorectal cancer cell lines but are uncommon [98]. However, decreased *TGFBR1* expression levels are frequently observed. In such cells, reconstitution of *TGFBR1* expression has been shown to decrease tumorigenesis. *TGFBR1**6A, a *TGFBR1* polymorphism that consists of a deletion of three alanines within a nine-alanine repeat at the 3' end of exon 1, results in an impairment of TGF-β-mediated anti-proliferative response and has been associated with increased cancer risk in several studies [99–101]. Liao et al. [102] recently published a meta-analysis of 32 studies including 13,662 cases and 14,147 controls. Overall, *TGFBR1**6A was significantly associated with cancer risk in all genetic models (for allelic effect: OR = 1.11; 95% CI = 1.03–1.21; for 6A/6A vs. 9A/9A: OR = 1.30; 95% CI = 1.01–1.69; for 9A/6A vs. 9A/9A: OR = 1.08; 95% CI = 1.01–1.15; for dominant model: OR = 1.08; 95% CI = 1.02–1.15; for recessive model: OR = 1.29; 95% CI = 1.00–1.68). Genotyping of germline and tumor DNA has shown that *TGFBR1*6A* is somatically acquired in approximately 2% of primary colon and head and neck tumors [103]. Exogenous TGF-β increases thymidine incorporation in breast cancer cells stably transfected with this variant and in colon cancer cells that endogenously harbor this allele [103], suggesting that *TGFBR1*6A* has oncogenic properties in established tumor cells. To determine the role of *TGFBR1*6A* in the tumor microenvironment, we microdissected tumors cells, stromal cell, and histologically "normal" epithelial cells adjacent to the tumor from individual with head and neck cancer and evidence of *TGFBR1*6A* somatic acquisition within the tumor tissue [104]. In head and neck cancer we found that the *TGFBR1*6A* allele was present in the tumor, immediately juxtaposed "normal" squamous epithelium and stroma as well as in adjacent true vocal cord epithelium and stroma. In colon cancer we found that the *TGFBR1*6A* allele had been somatically acquired by stromal cells up to 2 cm away from the tumor's edge. Importantly, we found higher *TGFBR1*6A/TGFBR1* allelic ratios in tumor tissues compared with stromal and epithelial tissues [104]. Hence, the amount of somatically acquired *TGFBR1*6A* allele in normal epithelial and stromal cells surrounding the tumor appears to be inversely proportional to the distance from the primary tumor, suggestive of tumor-centered centrifugal growth [104]. This provides strong support for the concept that *TGFBR1*6A* somatic acquisition is a critical event in the early stages of cancer development that is associated with field cancerization [104]. However, *TGFBR1*6A* is not a bona fide oncogene when transfected into NIH 3T3cells. Rather, its decreased TGF-β signaling capabilities result in reduced oncogenesis when compared with wild-type *TGFBR1* [105]. To test the hypothesis that constitutively decreased *TGFBR1* signaling contributes to colorectal cancer development, we generated a novel mouse model of *Tgfbr1* haploinsufficiency [106]. We found that *Tgfbr1* haploinsufficient mice crossed with mice carrying a mutation in the *Apc* tumor-suppressor gene develop two to three times more intestinal tumors than wild-type littermates. Importantly, invasive adenocarcinoma with features of human colon cancer is only identified among $Apc^{\mathrm{Min}/+};Tgfbr1^{+/-}$ mice, not among $Apc^{\mathrm{Min}/+};Tgfbr1^{+/+}$ mice [106]. These findings led us to study whether constitutively decreased *TGFBR1* expression is associated with human cancer. We recently reported that constitutively decreased *TGFRB1* expression is an inherited trait associated with significantly increased colorectal cancer risk [107]. We also found that somatically acquired mutations of the *TGFBR1* gene were significantly more common in the tumors of patients with constitutively decreased *TGFRB1* expression (11.5%) than in the tumors of patients without constitutively decreased *TGFRB1* expression (0%) [107]. The mechanism for the constitutively decreased expression is currently under investigation.

5   *SMAD* Mutations in Colorectal Cancer

Alterations in the genes encoding proteins playing a role in the downstream pathways of TGF-β signaling have been associated with a variety of cancers. *SMAD2* and *SMAD4* both map to chromosome 18q, a region commonly deleted in colon adenocarcinomas [90]. *SMAD4* also known as *DCC* is mutated in 16–38% of colorectal tumors [108–111]. *SMAD2* also located on 18q21 is lost in 6% of sporadic colon cancers [112]. *SMAD2* and *SMAD4* gene inactivation occurs by deletion of entire chromosomal segments, small deletions, frameshift, nonsense, and missense mutations [67]. As mentioned earlier, germline mutations in *SMAD4* have been noted in several juvenile polyposis families with an increased predisposition to colorectal cancer. Mice studies have shed more light into the role of *Smad4* in carcinogenesis supporting its role as a tumor suppressor. Homozygous loss of *Smad4* leads to death of mice in utero, but heterozygous mice are viable [113–115]. These mice develop gastric polyps which evolve into cancers at a late age. However, *Smad4*$^{+/-}$ mice do develop colorectal tumors but only in the context of a primed, *Apc*-defective genetic background [116, 117]. *Smad4* deletion in the intestinal epithelium does not lead to tumor formation in the mice but a deletion in the T-cell compartment leads to the formation of numerous gastrointestinal tumors with infiltration by plasma cells [81]. These data suggest that *Smad4* plays an important and complex role in the interaction between the immune system, stroma and the epithelium, a disruption of which contributes to colorectal carcinogenesis. Clinically, the loss of *SMAD4* is associated with late-stage colon cancer and metastatic disease [118, 119]. Low levels of SMAD4 protein or mRNA in the tumor are also predictive of a poor response to chemotherapy and significantly shorter survival when compared to patients with tumors expressing high levels of SMAD4 [120, 121].

SMAD3 mutations have been thought to be infrequent in cancers. Mutational analysis of 11 colorectal cancer cell lines revealed a novel missense mutation in *SMAD3* (R273H) in the SNU-769A cell line. This mutation led to inhibition of the translocation of SMAD3 to the nucleus and decrease in the activity of SMAD3 during TGF-β-induced transcriptional activation [98]. Genome-wide analysis of protein coding genes in breast and colorectal cancers revealed that *SMAD3* is mutated at a significantly higher frequency than the background mutation rate in these tumors [122]. *Smad3* mutant mice are viable and fertile but develop colorectal adenocarcinomas between 4 and 6 months of age [123]. These mice also enhance intestinal tumorigenesis with an increase in multiplicity and rapid onset of invasive adenocarcinomas when crossed with *Apc*$^{Min/+}$ mice [124]. However, two other *Smad3* mutant mice generated independently did not reveal a higher incidence of colorectal malignancies but exhibited functional defects in the immune system [125, 126]. A potential explanation for this discrepancy may be related to the interaction of the immune system with the environment. When *Smad3*$^{-/-}$ mice are maintained in *H. pylori*-free environment, they do not develop colon cancer for up to 9 months of age. But infection of these mice with *Helicobacter* spp. leads to development of colon cancer in 55–60% of animals [80]. When *Smad3*-deficient mice are crossed with mice deficient in both B and T lymphocytes (*Rag2*$^{-/-}$), the progeny have a higher incidence of *Helicobacter*-induced diffuse inflammation, and adenocarcinoma of the colon when compared with *Helicobacter*-infected *Smad3*$^{-/-}$ or *Rag2*$^{-/-}$ mice. In addition, adoptive transfer of wild-type T-regulatory cells provided significant protection against colorectal cancer in the double knockout mice [127].

This suggests that loss of *Smad3* may contribute to colon cancer development by a combination of altered T-regulatory cell function, increased pro-inflammatory cytokines, and anti-apoptotic proteins leading to increased proliferation in colonic tissues.

6 Bone Morphogenetic Protein Pathway

Bone morphogenetic proteins are members of the TGF-β superfamily of proteins. The signaling cascade is similar to that described in the TGF-β pathway, involving the activation of the type 2 receptor by the ligand. The activated type 2 receptor phosphorylates the type 1 receptor and ultimately leads to the release of R-SMADs, which complex with SMAD4 and modulates target gene expression. The R-SMADs of the BMP pathway are SMAD1, SMAD5, and SMAD8. Activation of the BMP pathway can be assayed by using antibodies specific to phosphorylated forms of SMAD1, SMAD5, and SMAD8. BMP signaling inhibits intestinal stem cell renewal through suppression of the Wnt-β-catenin pathway [128]. BMP signaling is also required for full maturation of secretory cell lineages, in the small intestine in vivo and may have a role in apoptosis of mature colonic epithelial cells [129]. As mentioned earlier in the chapter, germline mutations in the *BMPR1A* gene have been described in patients with juvenile polyposis syndrome. A role for the alteration of the BMP pathway in sporadic colorectal cancer is emerging. At the ligand level, BMP2, BMP3, and BMP7 have been found to be growth suppressive [129]. Downregulation of BMP3 was observed in 90% of colorectal cancer samples, in association with aberrant hypermethylation in the tumors and highly correlated with microsatellite instability. Approximately 76% of adenomas also exhibited downregulation of the promoter suggesting that silencing of BMP3 may be an early event in the progression of colorectal carcinogenesis via the serrated and the traditional pathways [130]. However, BMP7 was noted to be overexpressed at the mRNA and protein level in colonic tumor tissue when compared to normal tissue. Overexpression of BMP7 was associated with liver metastasis and poor prognosis [131]. Similarly, overexpression of BMP4, assessed by real-time RT-PCR and immunohistochemistry, was noted in late-stage adenocarcinomas and in tumors with liver metastasis when compared to normal tissue [132]. Interestingly, genome-wide association studies have revealed that SNP rs4444235 which is 9.4 kb from the transcription start site of BMP4 predisposes to colorectal cancer (odds ratio 1.11, 95% CI 1.08–1.15, $p = 8.1 \times 10^{-10}$) [32]. This association was significantly stronger in cases with microsatellite stable tumors compared with microsatellite unstable tumors.

It is possible that the BMP pathway may be inactivated during the transition from adenoma to carcinoma as almost 90% of adenomas have evidence of a functioning BMP pathway and loss of the pathway correlates with progression of adenoma to carcinoma [133]. The BMP pathway, assessed by nuclear staining of pSMAD1/5/8 expression, is inactivated in up to 70% of sporadic colorectal cancers.

The BMP receptor (BMPR2) expression is impaired in a majority of microsatellite unstable cancer cell lines. In addition, BMPR2 expression was significantly more frequently impaired in microsatellite unstable tumors than microsatellite stable tumors recapitulating the phenomenon seen with the type 2 TGF-β receptor (TGFBR2) [134].

7 SMAD Antagonists

SMAD6 and SMAD7 are inhibitory SMADs that negatively control TGF-β signaling in response to feedback loops and antagonistic signals [135]. SMAD6 competes with SMAD4 for binding to receptor-activated SMAD1, and SMAD7 recruits SMURF to TGF-β and BMP receptors for inactivation. Overexpression of SMAD7 and suppression of TGF-β signaling has been reported in endometrial carcinomas and thyroid follicular tumors [136, 137]. Interestingly, a recent genome-wide association study has shown that common alleles of *SMAD7* that lead to decreased SMAD7 mRNA expression are associated with colorectal cancer risk [31]. SMAD function is also directly inhibited by transcriptional repressors such as SKI and SNON (SKI-like). Deletions as well as amplification of *SKI* and *SKIL* have been reported in colorectal and esophageal cancers, raising the possibility that these genes act as oncogenes or tumor-suppressor genes depending on the context [138].

8 Future Directions

The recent exciting discoveries from genome-wide association studies in colorectal cancer have unearthed alterations at multiple levels in the TGF-β pathway, including BMP4, SMAD4, and SMAD7. At first glance, it seems that the risk of colorectal cancer with the inherited genomic loci is only slightly increased with an odds ratio less than 1.5. But, germline allele-specific expression in TGFBR1 [107] has been found to confer a substantially increased risk of colorectal cancer (odds ratio 8.7) even by conservative estimates. The findings need to be confirmed in larger studies and in different populations. Unlike most other human malignancies, we can screen for colorectal cancer effectively by fecal occult blood testing or colonoscopy. However, screening the entire population to identify early colon cancer is not a practical approach in terms of expense and availability of health-care workforce, and this practice may not benefit a large majority of the population. The immediate clinical application of the identification of high-risk genomic loci and allele-specific expression is that they can help us identify a group of individuals who are at a higher risk of developing colon cancer. Institution of thorough screening in such high-risk groups by screening individuals at an earlier age and/or more frequently than the general population may be a more effective approach.

The multiple pro-tumorigenic effects of the TGF-β pathway, enabling tumors to evade host immunity, facilitating invasion and metastasis make it a primary target for therapeutic interventions. However, the potential benefits of such a strategy have to be weighed against the potential complications associated with the inhibition of a pathway which has important roles in the maintenance of tissue homeostasis. A better understanding of this complex pathway with a focus on delineating the pro-tumorigenic effects and mechanisms in specific tumor types and at different phases of carcinogenesis and cancer progression is essential.

Acknowledgments This work is supported by grants R01 CA108741, R01 CA112520, R01 137000, and P60 AR048098 from NIH.

References

1. Jemal A, Siegel R, Ward E et al (2009) Cancer statistics, 2009. CA: A Cancer Journal for Clinicians, 59(4):225–249
2. Moertel C, Fleming TR, Macdonald JS, Mailliard JA (1995) Fluorouracil plus levamisole as effective adjuvant therapy after resection of stage III colon carcinoma: a final report. Ann Int Med 122:321–326
3. Hurwitz H, Fehrenbacher L, Novotny W et al (2004) Bevacizumab plus irinotecan, fluorouracil, and leucovorin for metastatic colorectal cancer. N Engl J Med 350: 2335–2342
4. Fuchs CS, Giovannucci EL, Colditz GA, Hunter DJ, Speizer FE, Willett WC (1994) A prospective study of family history and the risk of colorectal cancer. N Engl J Med 331:1669–1674
5. Johns LE, Houlston RS (2001) A systematic review and meta-analysis of familial colorectal cancer risk. Am J Gastroenterol 96:2992–3003
6. Butterworth AS, Higgins JP, Pharoah P (2006) Relative and absolute risk of colorectal cancer for individuals with a family history: a meta-analysis. Eur J Cancer 42:216–227
7. Lichtenstein P, Holm NV, Verkasalo PK et al (2000) Environmental and heritable factors in the causation of cancer – analyses of cohorts of twins from Sweden, Denmark, and Finland. N Engl J Med 343:78–85
8. Bisgaard ML, Fenger K, Bulow S, Niebuhr E, Mohr J (1994) Familial adenomatous polyposis (FAP): frequency, penetrance, and mutation rate. Hum Mutat 3:121–125
9. Lynch HT, de la Chapelle A (2003) Hereditary colorectal cancer. N Engl J Med 348: 919–932
10. Laken SJ, Petersen GM, Gruber SB et al (1997) Familial colorectal cancer in Ashkenazim due to a hypermutable tract in APC. Nat Genet 17:79–83
11. Rozen P, Shomrat R, Strul H et al (1999) Prevalence of the I1307K APC gene variant in Israeli Jews of differing ethnic origin and risk for colorectal cancer. Gastroenterology 116:54–57
12. Rustgi AK (2007) The genetics of hereditary colon cancer. Genes Dev 21:2525–2538
13. Foulkes WD (2008) Inherited susceptibility to common cancers. N Engl J Med 359: 2143–2153
14. Lynch HT, Lynch JF, Lynch PM, Attard T (2008) Hereditary colorectal cancer syndromes: molecular genetics, genetic counseling, diagnosis and management. Fam Cancer 7:27–39
15. Al-Tassan N, Chmiel NH, Maynard J et al (2002) Inherited variants of MYH associated with somatic G:C–>T:A mutations in colorectal tumors. Nat Genet 30:227–232
16. Avezzu A, Agostini M, Pucciarelli S et al (2008) The role of MYH gene in genetic predisposition to colorectal cancer: another piece of the puzzle. Cancer Lett 268:308–313

17. Colebatch A, Hitchins M, Williams R, Meagher A, Hawkins NJ, Ward RL (2006) The role of MYH and microsatellite instability in the development of sporadic colorectal cancer. Br J Cancer 95:1239–1243

18. Croitoru ME, Cleary SP, Di Nicola N et al (2004) Association between biallelic and monoallelic germline MYH gene mutations and colorectal cancer risk. J Natl Cancer Inst 96:1631–1634

19. Enholm S, Hienonen T, Suomalainen A et al (2003) Proportion and phenotype of MYH-associated colorectal neoplasia in a population-based series of Finnish colorectal cancer patients. Am J Pathol 163:827–832

20. Kambara T, Whitehall VL, Spring KJ et al (2004) Role of inherited defects of MYH in the development of sporadic colorectal cancer. Genes Chromosomes Cancer 40:1–9

21. Wang L, Baudhuin LM, Boardman LA et al (2004) MYH mutations in patients with attenuated and classic polyposis and with young-onset colorectal cancer without polyps. Gastroenterology 127:9–16

22. Zhou XL, Djureinovic T, Werelius B, Lindmark G, Sun XF, Lindblom A (2005) Germline mutations in the MYH gene in Swedish familial and sporadic colorectal cancer. Genet Test 9:147–151

23. Farrington SM, Tenesa A, Barnetson R et al (2005) Germline susceptibility to colorectal cancer due to base-excision repair gene defects. Am J Hum Genet 77:112–119

24. Lubbe SJ, Di Bernardo MC, Chandler IP, Houlston RS (2009) Clinical implications of the colorectal cancer risk associated with MUTYH mutation. J Clin Oncol 27:3975–3980

25. Lipton L, Halford SE, Johnson V et al (2003) Carcinogenesis in MYH-associated polyposis follows a distinct genetic pathway. Cancer Res 63:7595–7599

26. Poulsen ML, Bisgaard ML (2008) MUTYH associated polyposis (MAP). Curr Genomics 9:420–435

27. Kemp Z, Thirlwell C, Sieber O, Silver A, Tomlinson I (2004) An update on the genetics of colorectal cancer. Hum Mol Genet 13:R177–R185

28. Zanke BW, Greenwood CM, Rangrej J et al (2007) Genome-wide association scan identifies a colorectal cancer susceptibility locus on chromosome 8q24. Nat Genet 39:989–994

29. Tomlinson I, Webb E, Carvajal-Carmona L et al (2007) A genome-wide association scan of tag SNPs identifies a susceptibility variant for colorectal cancer at 8q24.21. Nat Genet 39:984–988

30. Jaeger E, Webb E, Howarth K et al (2008) Common genetic variants at the CRAC1 (HMPS) locus on chromosome 15q13.3 influence colorectal cancer risk. Nat Genet 40:26–28

31. Broderick P, Carvajal-Carmona L, Pittman AM et al (2007) A genome-wide association study shows that common alleles of SMAD7 influence colorectal cancer risk. Nat Genet 39:1315–1317

32. Houlston RS, Webb E, Broderick P et al (2008) Meta-analysis of genome-wide association data identifies four new susceptibility loci for colorectal cancer. Nat Genet 40: 1426–1435

33. Tenesa A, Farrington SM, Prendergast JG et al (2008) Genome-wide association scan identifies a colorectal cancer susceptibility locus on 11q23 and replicates risk loci at 8q24 and 18q21. Nat Genet 40:631–637

34. Lee IM, Paffenbarger RS Jr (1992) Quetelet's index and risk of colon cancer in college alumni. J Natl Cancer Inst 84:1326–1331

35. Calle EE, Rodriguez C, Walker-Thurmond K, Thun MJ (2003) Overweight, obesity, and mortality from cancer in a prospectively studied cohort of U.S. adults. N Engl J Med 348:1625–1638

36. Macinnis RJ, English DR, Hopper JL, Haydon AM, Gertig DM, Giles GG (2004) Body size and composition and colon cancer risk in men. Cancer Epidemiol Biomarkers Prev 13:553–559

37. Pischon T, Lahmann PH, Boeing H et al (2006) Body size and risk of colon and rectal cancer in the European prospective investigation into cancer and nutrition (EPIC). J Natl Cancer Inst 98:920–931

38. Larsson SC, Wolk A (2007) Obesity and colon and rectal cancer risk: a meta-analysis of prospective studies. Am J Clin Nutr 86:556–565
39. Wei EK, Giovannucci E, Fuchs CS, Willett WC, Mantzoros CS (2005) Low plasma adiponectin levels and risk of colorectal cancer in men: a prospective study. J Natl Cancer Inst 97:1688–1694
40. Wei EK, Ma J, Pollak MN et al (2005) A prospective study of C-peptide, insulin-like growth factor-I, insulin-like growth factor binding protein-1, and the risk of colorectal cancer in women. Cancer Epidemiol Biomarkers Prev 14:850–855
41. Giovannucci E, Pollak MN, Platz EA et al (2000) A prospective study of plasma insulin-like growth factor-1 and binding protein-3 and risk of colorectal neoplasia in women. Cancer Epidemiol Biomarkers Prev 9:345–349
42. Ma J, Giovannucci E, Pollak M et al (2004) A prospective study of plasma C-peptide and colorectal cancer risk in men. J Natl Cancer Inst 96:546–553
43. Sandhu MS, Dunger DB, Giovannucci EL (2002) Insulin, insulin-like growth factor-I (IGF-I), IGF binding proteins, their biologic interactions, and colorectal cancer. J Natl Cancer Inst 94:972–980
44. Kaklamani VG, Sadim M, Hsi A et al (2008) Variants of the adiponectin and adiponectin receptor 1 genes and breast cancer risk. Cancer Res 68:3178–3184
45. Carvajal-Carmona LG, Spain S, The CORGI Consortium et al (2009) Common variation at the adiponectin locus is not associated with colorectal cancer risk in the UK. Hum Mol Genet 18:1889–1892
46. Noffsinger AE (2009) Serrated polyps and colorectal cancer: new pathway to malignancy. Annu Rev Pathol 4:343–364
47. Castells A (2008) MYH-associated polyposis: adenomas and hyperplastic polyps, partners in crime? Gastroenterology 135:1857–1859
48. Wynter CV, Walsh MD, Higuchi T, Leggett BA, Young J, Jass JR (2004) Methylation patterns define two types of hyperplastic polyp associated with colorectal cancer. Gut 53:573–580
49. Nagasaka T, Sasamoto H, Notohara K et al (2004) Colorectal cancer with mutation in BRAF, KRAS, and wild-type with respect to both oncogenes showing different patterns of DNA methylation. J Clin Oncol 22:4584–4594
50. Kumar K, Brim H, Giardiello F et al (2009) Distinct BRAF (V600E) and KRAS mutations in high microsatellite instability sporadic colorectal cancer in African Americans. Clin Cancer Res 15:1155–1161
51. Samowitz WS, Albertsen H, Sweeney C et al (2006) Association of smoking, CpG island methylator phenotype, and V600E BRAF mutations in colon cancer. J Natl Cancer Inst 98:1731–1738
52. Ajioka Y, Watanabe H, Jass JR, Yokota Y, Kobayashi M, Nishikura K (1998) Infrequent K-ras codon 12 mutation in serrated adenomas of human colorectum. Gut 42:680–684
53. Sawyer EJ, Hanby AM, Rowan AJ et al (2002) The Wnt pathway, epithelial-stromal interactions, and malignant progression in phyllodes tumours. J Pathol 196:437–444
54. O'Brien MJ, Yang S, Mack C et al (2006) Comparison of microsatellite instability, CpG island methylation phenotype, BRAF and KRAS status in serrated polyps and traditional adenomas indicates separate pathways to distinct colorectal carcinoma end points. Am J Surg Pathol 30:1491–1501
55. O'Brien MJ, Yang S, Clebanoff JL et al (2004) Hyperplastic (serrated) polyps of the colorectum: relationship of CpG island methylator phenotype and K-ras mutation to location and histologic subtype. Am J Surg Pathol 28:423–434
56. Yang S, Farraye FA, Mack C, Posnik O, O'Brien MJ (2004) BRAF and KRAS Mutations in hyperplastic polyps and serrated adenomas of the colorectum: relationship to histology and CpG island methylation status. Am J Surg Pathol 28:1452–1459
57. Jass JR, Baker K, Zlobec I et al (2006) Advanced colorectal polyps with the molecular and morphological features of serrated polyps and adenomas: concept of a 'fusion' pathway to colorectal cancer. Histopathology 49:121–131

58. Chan TL, Zhao W, Leung SY, Yuen ST (2003) BRAF and KRAS mutations in colorectal hyperplastic polyps and serrated adenomas. Cancer Res 63:4878–4881

59. Spring KJ, Zhao ZZ, Karamatic R et al (2006) High prevalence of sessile serrated adenomas with BRAF mutations: a prospective study of patients undergoing colonoscopy. Gastroenterology 131:1400–1407

60. Rajagopalan H, Bardelli A, Lengauer C, Kinzler KW, Vogelstein B, Velculescu VE (2002) Tumorigenesis: RAF/RAS oncogenes and mismatch-repair status. Nature 418:934

61. Brosens LAA, van Hattem A, Hylind LM et al (2007) Risk of colorectal cancer in juvenile polyposis. Gut 56:965–967

62. Howe JR, Ringold JC, Summers RW, Mitros FA, Nishimura DY, Stone EM (1998) A gene for familial juvenile polyposis maps to chromosome 18q21.1. Am J Hum Genet 62:1129–1136

63. Howe JR, Roth S, Ringold JC et al (1998) Mutations in the SMAD4/DPC4 gene in juvenile polyposis. Science 280:1086–1088

64. Sweet K, Willis J, Zhou XP et al (2005) Molecular classification of patients with unexplained hamartomatous and hyperplastic polyposis. JAMA 294:2465–2473

65. Howe JR, Haidle JL, Lal G et al (2007) ENG mutations in MADH4/BMPR1A mutation negative patients with juvenile polyposis. Clin Genet 71:91–92

66. Grady WM, Carethers JM (2008) Genomic and epigenetic instability in colorectal cancer pathogenesis. Gastroenterology 135:1079–1099

67. Massague J, Blain SW, Lo RS (2000) TGFbeta signaling in growth control, cancer, and heritable disorders. Cell 103:295–309

68. Shi Y, Massague J (2003) Mechanisms of TGF-beta signaling from cell membrane to the nucleus. Cell 113:685–700

69. Goumans MJ, Valdimarsdottir G, Itoh S et al (2003) Activin receptor-like kinase (ALK)1 is an antagonistic mediator of lateral TGF[beta]/ALK5 signaling. Mol Cell 12:817–828

70. Imamura T, Takase M, Nishihara A et al (1997) Smad6 inhibits signalling by the tgf-beta superfamily. Nature 389:622–626

71. Ebisawa T, Fukuchi M, Murakami G et al (2001) Smurf1 interacts with transforming growth factor-beta type I receptor through Smad7 and induces receptor degradation. J Biol Chem 276:12477–12480

72. Shi W, Sun C, He B et al (2004) GADD34-PP1c recruited by Smad7 dephosphorylates TGFbeta type I receptor. J Cell Biol 164:291–300

73. Massague J (1998) TGF-beta signal transduction. Annu Rev Biochem 67:753–791

74. Massague J (2008) TGFbeta in Cancer. Cell 134:215–230

75. Kim YS, Yi YS, Choi SG, Kim SJ (1999) Development of TGF-beta resistance during malignant progression [review]. Arch Pharm Res 22:1–8

76. Grady WM, Myeroff LL, Swinler SE et al (1999) Mutational inactivation of transforming growth factor beta receptor type II in microsatellite stable colon cancers. Cancer Res 59: 320–324

77. Derynck R, Akhurst RJ, Balmain A (2001) TGF-beta signaling in tumor suppression and cancer progression. Nat Genet 29:117–129

78. Bhowmick NA, Chytil A, Plieth D et al (2004) TGF-{beta} signaling in fibroblasts modulates the oncogenic potential of adjacent epithelia. Science 303:848–851

79. Cheng N, Chytil A, Shyr Y, Joly A, Moses HL (2008) Transforming growth factor-{beta} signaling-deficient fibroblasts enhance hepatocyte growth factor signaling in mammary carcinoma cells to promote scattering and invasion. Mol Cancer Res 6:1521–1533

80. Maggio-Price L, Treuting P, Zeng W, Tsang M, Bielefeldt-Ohmann H, Iritani BM (2006) Helicobacter infection is required for inflammation and colon cancer in Smad3-deficient mice. Cancer Res 66:828–838

81. Kim BG, Li C, Qiao W et al (2006) Smad4 signalling in T cells is required for suppression of gastrointestinal cancer. Nature 441:1015–1019

82. Shipitsin M, Campbell LL, Argani P et al (2007) Molecular definition of breast tumor heterogeneity. Cancer Cell 11:259–273

83. Thiery JP (2003) Epithelial-mesenchymal transitions in development and pathologies. Curr Opin Cell Biol 15:740–746

84. Derynck R, Akhurst RJ (2007) Differentiation plasticity regulated by TGF-[beta] family proteins in development and disease. Nat Cell Biol 9:1000–1004

85. Mani SA, Guo W, Liao MJ et al (2008) The epithelial-mesenchymal transition generates cells with properties of stem cells. Cell 133:704–715

86. Thuault S, Valcourt U, Petersen M, Manfioletti G, Heldin CH, Moustakas A (2006) Transforming growth factor-{beta} employs HMGA2 to elicit epithelial-mesenchymal transition. J Cell Biol 174:175–183

87. Thuault S, Tan EJ, Peinado H, Cano A, Heldin CH, Moustakas A (2008) HMGA2 and Smads co-regulate SNAIL1 expression during induction of epithelial-to-mesenchymal transition. J Biol Chem 283:33437–33446

88. Ozdamar B, Bose R, Barrios-Rodiles M, Wang HR, Zhang Y, Wrana JL (2005) Regulation of the polarity protein Par6 by TGFbeta receptors controls epithelial cell plasticity. Science 307:1603–1609

89. Seton-Rogers SE, Lu Y, Hines LM et al (2004) Cooperation of the ErbB2 receptor and trans-forming growth factor beta in induction of migration and invasion in mammary epithelial cells. Proc Natl Acad Sci USA 101:1257–1262

90. Grady WM, Markowitz SD (2002) Genetic and epigenetic alterations in colon cancer. Annu Rev Genom Hum Genet 3:101–128

91. Takayama T, Miyanishi K, Hayashi T, Sato Y, Niitsu Y (2006) Colorectal cancer: genetics of development and metastasis. J Gastroenterol 41:185–192

92. Parsons R, Myeroff LL, Liu B et al (1995) Microsatellite instability and mutations of the transforming growth factor beta type II receptor gene in colorectal cancer. Cancer Res 55:5548–5550

93. Ilyas M, Efstathiou JA, Straub J, Kim HC, Bodmer WF (1999) Transforming growth fac-tor beta stimulation of colorectal cancer cell lines: type II receptor bypass and changes in adhesion molecule expression. Proc Natl Acad Sci USA 96:3087–3091

94. Grady WM, Willis JE, Trobridge P et al (2006) Proliferation and Cdk4 expression in microsatellite unstable colon cancers with TGFBR2 mutations. Int J Cancer 118:600–608

95. Watanabe T, Wu TT, Catalano PJ et al (2001) Molecular predictors of survival after adjuvant chemotherapy for colon cancer. N Engl J Med 344:1196–1206

96. Samowitz WS, Curtin K, Leppert MF, Slattery ML (2002) The prognostic implications of BAX and TGF[BETA]RII mutations in colon cancers with microsatellite instability. Mod Pathol 15:143A

97. Samowitz WS, Curtin K, Neuhausen S, Schaffer D, Slattery ML (2002) Prognostic implica-tions of BAX and TGFBRII mutations in colon cancers with microsatellite instability. Genes Chromosomes Cancer 35:368–371

98. Ku JL, Park SH, Yoon KA et al (2007) Genetic alterations of the TGF-beta signaling pathway in colorectal cancer cell lines: a novel mutation in Smad3 associated with the inactivation of TGF-beta-induced transcriptional activation. Cancer Lett 247:283–292

99. Kaklamani VG, Hou N Bian Y et al (2003) TGFBR1*6A and cancer risk: a meta-analysis of seven case-control studies. J Clin Oncol 21:3236–3243

100. Pasche B, Kaklamani VG, Hou N et al (2004) TGFBR1*6A and cancer: a meta-analysis of 12 case-control studies. J Clin Oncol 22:756–758

101. Zhang HT, Zhao J, Zheng SY, Chen XF (2005) Is TGFBR1*6A really associated with increased risk of cancer? J Clin Oncol 23:7743–7744

102. Liao RY, Mao C, Qiu LX, Ding H, Chen Q, Pan HF (2009) TGFBR1*6A/9A polymor-phism and cancer risk: a meta-analysis of 13,662 cases and 14,147 controls. Mol Biol Rep (published online November 1, 2009)

103. Pasche B, Knobloch TJ, Bian Y et al (2005) Somatic acquisition and signaling of TGFBR1*6A in cancer. JAMA 294:1634–1646

104. Bian Y, Knobloch TJ, Sadim M et al (2007) Somatic acquisition of TGFBR1*6A by epithelial and stromal cells during head and neck and colon cancer development. Hum Mol Genet 16:3128–3135
105. Rosman DS, Phukan S, Huang CC, Pasche B (2008) TGFBR1*6A enhances the migration and invasion of MCF-7 breast cancer cells through RhoA activation. Cancer Res 68: 1319–1328
106. Zeng Q, Phukan S, Xu Y et al (2009) Tgfbr1 haploinsufficiency is a potent modifier of colorectal cancer development. Cancer Res 69:678–686
107. Valle L, Serena-Acedo T, Liyanarachchi S et al (2008) Germline allele-specific expression of TGFBR1 confers an increased risk of colorectal cancer. Science 321:1361–1365
108. Thiagalingam S, Lengauer C, Leach FS et al (1996) Evaluation of candidate tumour suppressor genes on chromosome 18 in colorectal cancers. Nat Genet 13:343–346
109. Takagi Y, Kohmura H, Futamura M et al (1996) Somatic alterations of the dpc4 gene in human colorectal cancers in vivo. Gastroenterology 111:1369–1372
110. Ando T, Sugai T, Habano W, Jiao YF, Suzuki K (2005) Analysis of SMAD4/DPC4 gene alterations in multiploid colorectal carcinomas. J Gastroenterol 40:708–715
111. Salovaara R, Roth S, Loukola A et al (2002) Frequent loss of SMAD4/DPC4 protein in colorectal cancers. Gut 51:56–59
112. Eppert K, Scherer SW, Ozcelik H et al (1996) Madr2 maps to 18q21 and encodes a tgfbeta-regulated mad-related protein that is functionally mutated in colorectal carcinoma. Cell 86:543–552
113. Yang X, Li CL, Xu XL, Deng CX (1998) The tumor suppressor smad4/dpc4 is essential for epiblast proliferation and mesoderm induction in mice. Proc Natl Acad Sci USA 95: 3667–3672
114. Weinstein M, Yang X, Deng C (2000) Functions of mammalian Smad genes as revealed by targeted gene disruption in mice. Cytokine Growth Factor Rev 11:49–58
115. Mishra L, Shetty K, Tang Y, Stuart A, Byers SW (2005) The role of TGF-beta and Wnt signaling in gastrointestinal stem cells and cancer. Oncogene 24:5775–5789
116. Takaku K, Oshima M, Miyoshi H, Matsui M, Seldin MF, Taketo MM (1998) Intestinal tumorigenesis in compound mutant mice of both dpc4 (Smad4) and apc genes. Cell 92:645–656
117. Kitamura T, Kometani K, Hashida H et al (2007) SMAD4-deficient intestinal tumors recruit CCR1[+] myeloid cells that promote invasion. Nat Genet 39:467–475
118. Maitra A, Krueger JE, Tascilar M et al (2000) Carcinoid tumors of the extrahepatic bile ducts: a study of seven cases. Am J Surg Pathol 24:1501–1510
119. Isaksson-Mettavainio M, Palmqvist R, Forssell J, Stenling R, Oberg A (2006) SMAD4/DPC4 expression and prognosis in human colorectal cancer. Anticancer Res 26:507–510
120. Alazzouzi H, Alhopuro P, Salovaara R et al (2005) SMAD4 as a prognostic marker in colorectal cancer. Clin Cancer Res 11:2606–2611
121. Boulay JL, Mild G, Lowy A et al (2002) SMAD4 is a predictive marker for 5-fluorouracil-based chemotherapy in patients with colorectal cancer. Br J Cancer 87:630–634
122. Sjoblom T, Jones S, Wood LD et al (2006) The consensus coding sequences of human breast and colorectal cancers. Science 314:268–274
123. Zhu YA, Richardson JA, Parada LF, Graff JM (1998) Smad3 mutant mice develop metastatic colorectal cancer. Cell 94:703–714
124. Sodir NM, Chen X, Park R et al (2006) Smad3 deficiency promotes tumorigenesis in the distal colon of ApcMin/+ mice. Cancer Res 66:8430–8438
125. Datto MB, Frederick JP, Pan LH, Borton AJ, Zhuang Y, Wang XF (1999) Targeted disruption of Smad3 reveals an essential role in transforming growth factor beta-mediated signal transduction. Mol Cell Biol 19:2495–2504

126. Yang X, Letterio JJ, Lechleider RJ et al (1999) Targeted disruption of SMAD3 results in impaired mucosal immunity and diminished T cell responsiveness to TGF-beta. EMBO J 18:1280–1291
127. Maggio-Price L, Treuting P, Bielefeldt-Ohmann H et al (2009) Bacterial infection of Smad3/Rag2 double-null mice with transforming growth factor-beta dysregulation as a model for studying inflammation-associated colon cancer. Am J Pathol 174:317–329
128. He XC, Zhang J, Tong WG et al (2004) BMP signaling inhibits intestinal stem cell self-renewal through suppression of Wnt-[beta]-catenin signaling. Nat Genet 36:1117–1121
129. Hardwick JC, Kodach LL, Offerhaus GJ, van den Brink GR (2008) Bone morphogenetic protein signalling in colorectal cancer. Nat Rev Cancer 8:806–812
130. Loh K, Chia JA, Greco S et al (2008) Bone morphogenic protein 3 inactivation is an early and frequent event in colorectal cancer development. Genes Chromosomes Cancer 47:449–460
131. Motoyama K, Tanaka F, Kosaka Y et al (2008) Clinical significance of BMP7 in human colorectal cancer. Ann Surg Oncol 15:1530–1537
132. Deng H, Ravikumar TS, Yang WL (2009) Overexpression of bone morphogenetic protein 4 enhances the invasiveness of Smad4-deficient human colorectal cancer cells. Cancer Lett 281:220–231
133. Kodach LL, Wiercinska E, de Miranda NF et al (2008) The bone morphogenetic protein pathway is inactivated in the majority of sporadic colorectal cancers. Gastroenterology 134:1332–1341
134. Kodach LL, Wiercinska E, de Miranda NF et al (2008) The bone morphogenetic protein pathway is inactivated in the majority of sporadic colorectal cancers. Gastroenterology 134:1332–1341
135. Massague J, Seoane J, Wotton D (2005) Smad transcription factors. Genes Dev 19:2783–2810
136. Cerutti JM, Ebina KN, Matsuo SE, Martins L, Maciel RM, Kimura ET (2003) Expression of Smad4 and Smad7 in human thyroid follicular carcinoma cell lines. J Endocrinol Invest 26:516–521
137. Dowdy SC, Mariani A, Reinholz MM et al (2005) Overexpression of the TGF-beta antagonist Smad7 in endometrial cancer. Gynecol Oncol 96:368–373
138. Zhu Q, Krakowski AR, Dunham EE et al (2007) Dual role of SnoN in mammalian tumorigenesis. Mol Cell Biol 27:324–339

Index

Note: The letters 'f' and 't' followed by the locators refer to figures and tables respectively.

B. Pasche (ed.), *Cancer Genetics*, Cancer Treatment and Research 155,
DOI 10.1007/978-1-4419-6033-7, © Springer Science+Business Media, LLC 2010

GPSR Compliance
The European Union's (EU) General Product Safety Regulation (GPSR) is a set
of rules that requires consumer products to be safe and our obligations to
ensure this.

If you have any concerns about our products, you can contact us on

ProductSafety@springernature.com

In case Publisher is established outside the EU, the EU authorized
representative is:

Springer Nature Customer Service Center GmbH
Europaplatz 3
69115 Heidelberg, Germany